FAT

From Desperation to Relief

Laura Dolan-Hayes

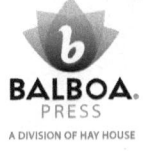

BALBOA.
PRESS

A DIVISION OF HAY HOUSE

Balboa Press books may be ordered through booksellers or by contacting:

Balboa Press
A Division of Hay House
1663 Liberty Drive
Bloomington, IN 47403
www.balboapress.com
1-(877) 407-4847

Because of the dynamic nature of the Internet, any web addresses or links contained in this book may have changed since publication and may no longer be valid. The views expressed in this work are solely those of the author and do not necessarily reflect the views of the publisher, and the publisher hereby disclaims any responsibility for them.

The author of this book does not dispense medical advice or prescribe the use of any technique as a form of treatment for physical, emotional, or medical problems without the advice of a physician, either directly or indirectly. The intent of the author is only to offer information of a general nature to help you in your quest for emotional and spiritual well-being. In the event you use any of the information in this book for yourself, which is your constitutional right, the author and the publisher assume no responsibility for your actions.

Any people depicted in stock imagery provided by Thinkstock are models, and such images are being used for illustrative purposes only.
Certain stock imagery © Thinkstock.

Print information available on the last page.

ISBN: 978-1-4525-4877-7 (sc)
ISBN: 978-1-4525-4876-0 (e)

Library of Congress Control Number: 2012904890

Balboa Press rev. date: 2/9/2016

Also by Laura Dolan-Hayes

Unemployed: How Desperation Led Me to the Worst Job Ever

To my belly: I'm so sorry, please forgive me

Preface

It is vitally important that you read this preface before you begin reading the book itself. The design of this book is one where you actually go on a six year journey of self-discovery with me when it comes to the topic of weight. I make some very bold statements in the beginning of the book, and then you follow me as I journal my progress toward defaulting back to my natural thinness. You will bear witness to the struggle I go through in letting go of popular notions about weight and weight control. I have many "ah ha" moments where I think I have figured everything out, just to be thwarted again. When you read one of those "ah ha" moments and there are pages to follow, I still had a way to go until gaining complete understanding. Please refrain from doing anything I do in the book until you have finished reading it completely.

The reason I chose to write the book this way, rather than just coming up with my conclusions and presenting them is because I want to show you how miserably I struggled, and for how long I struggled to come to the understanding that all the control we will ever need or want, lies in the power of our thoughts. I have done almost no editing during the text where I'm treating this book like my personal journal. These are my real thoughts and feelings. These are my real "light bulb" moments. What I want you to know more than anything is that like you, I have struggled and fought with my weight, and even in light of having some intellectual understanding that what we're doing is downright crazy, I had to think myself out of the insanity. You will bear witness to the struggle of marrying my intellectual understanding with the emotional side which has been abused by misinformation for the last thirty-six years.

Enjoy the story and enjoy the ride, but please don't put any "advice" I suggest in the book into play until you get to the conclusion. Also, please don't jump to the end because the ending will make no sense without going on the full journey with me. I know many of you will see yourselves in my words, and this is why I want you to read the book completely before taking any advice from me at all.

Hey it's Laura again. When you see italic writing at the top of the chapter or entry, this is the recovered me talking. I'm just giving you some warning at the top of the page that indicates that I'm probably still struggling pretty hard, or I may be contradicting what I said the chapter before. In any event, it's just a head's up so you don't suffer too much whiplash as I think myself to the truth. I apologize in advance for the crazy ride you are about to go on.

Acknowledgements

I would like to thank the following people who were instrumental in helping me get this book written. First I would like to thank me, because without me, this book wouldn't have been written, and that would have been a shame.

A big thank you goes out to my mother-in-law Terry for your support. You are the only person who understood the gravity of what I was writing about, and whole heartedly supported my theory. Without your help this book would not have sped onto the market the way it did.

Thank you to my husband Ken. Although you didn't know I was writing this book, I want to thank you for your support. You encouraged me to work in our business together, which has given me the gift of time to write this book. I couldn't be more thankful for your kindness of spirit and your generosity.

I would like to thank Rhonda Byrne, author of *The Secret* and her brief story of how she went back to her default perfect natural weight. It sent me on my own personal mission of understanding that I am so happily sharing with the world today.

Thank you to my friend Carrie Chavers-Wills for suspending disbelief and listening to me as I agonized with the struggle. I know I gave you many cases of virtual whiplash, but in the end it was worth it.

Thank you to my BFF Lori Jeffers. Having lived through your gastric bypass and being witness to the barbaric fallout, only makes the work I'm doing in this book more important. Thank you.

I want to say a special thank you to my new favorite medical doctor Munirih Tahzib, MD. I had some medical fallout after finally turning my back on old beliefs. Dr. Tahzib restored my faith in medicine by acknowledging how powerful the mind/body connection is, and that I am truly on the right track. Thank you so much for helping me Dr. Tahzib!

I am forever grateful to Robert Comeau, English professor at Union County College in Cranford, New Jersey. Thank you for the encouragement you gave me about my writing. Thank you for saying that if I didn't choose writing as a profession, I have chosen the wrong career. Those words mean more to me than you will ever know.

Thank you to my publisher Balboa Press for your speed and professionalism in getting this book to market.

Contents

Chapter 1

My Personal Odyssey with Weight

Hi it's me Laura...if you skipped the Preface and just launched to Chapter 1, please go back to the Preface for a minute. It's really short, but I need you to read it before you start the book. It's important. Thanks.

A s I WRITE THE FIRST WORDS in this book, it is June 3, 2010 and I'm sitting at my dining room table at a whopping one hundred and eighty four pounds. I have known for six months that I wanted to write the ultimate book on leveraging the Law of Attraction, or "what you think is what you get" to return back to a normal healthy weight, but I discovered that I was about as immersed into the Culture of Fat as anyone can be. For the last six months, through journaling, I have had long and often painful discussions with myself, and looking back I can understand why no effort to be thin was working.

One of the things I'm beginning to understand is that controlling my weight is a big effort and requires too much of my thought and time. It is stress and struggle on a nearly constant basis.

On my way out to my car this morning, as I walked through the fresh, dewy grass, I remembered a line from the book *The Secret*. The line says "The grass does not strain to grow." That revelation set me on a new thought path.

I have deliberately used The Law of Attraction to manifest many things in my life. I do it purposefully and I get amazing results. The Law of Attraction simply states that you get what you think most about. As a result my relationships are greatly improved. I am attracting new friends into my life. My first book is in the edit process. All of these things are a direct result of my asking the Universe for specific things and then receiving them. But I look at myself and wonder why I'm not at my perfect weight? I've asked to be returned to my perfect weight and I'm still one hundred and eighty four pounds.

This morning I realized that there are many things at play here, and today is the first day my body will begin to return to its perfect size, because I have changed my thinking and I have stopped struggling against fat. For the last thirty years I have tried to control my weight, and it hasn't worked out very well for me. All these years I have been coming up with a plan to lose the weight. I got sucked into the "how" of losing weight. One of my plans was to walk everywhere I could. My rationalization was that when I was a teenager I walked everywhere, and I was naturally thin. What I failed to consider was that after the age of eighteen I drove everywhere and continued to be naturally thin. Then I thought about my childhood. No kids were fat because we played outside all of the time. We were riding bikes and running around the neighborhood, we played hop scotch and hula hoop, and jumped rope. What I failed to consider was that in the wintertime here in New Jersey it was too cold to go outside and play. From November to April we were fairly sedentary and yet I remained perfectly naturally thin.

Just this morning I realized that I was clearly spending too much time and energy on the topic of losing weight. This struggle is useless, and it's keeping the weight on me rather than allowing me to return to my natural weight naturally. When I was a teen, it wasn't the walking that kept me thin, it was me assuming I was thin that kept me thin. When I was a child, it wasn't the bike riding or the hop scotch that kept me thin, it was the lack of fat thoughts that kept me thin.

What I want to talk about is my dysfunctional relationship with fat. Fat and I were first introduced when I was eleven years old, in 1970. At that time the world-wide fat panic was in its infancy. At the age of eleven I had chunked up a little bit and my mother panicked. She took me to the doctor who put me on an Atkins type diet. I did get thin again, but not because of the diet, but because I grew tall. It wasn't until I became a mother myself that I realized my kids would chunk up right before they had a growth spurt. So at the tender age of eleven the "fat" word had been introduced into my psyche where it has taken up permanent residence for the last forty years. Throughout junior high I chunked up and leaned out many times until I came out the other side at a perfect one hundred and eighteen pounds.

I maintained that weight until I got married at twenty-two years old, and began adopting the fat myths. I gained four "newlywed" pounds. I managed to maintain the one hundred and twenty-two pounds until I got pregnant with my daughter. After giving birth I was one hundred and forty-one pounds, because it's hard to lose weight after you have a baby. I yo-yo dieted for the next five years until I was one hundred and forty four pounds when I got pregnant with my son. After he was born, twenty-one years ago, I was in the one sixties and after that much of my weight struggles have become a blur. I have gone on so many diets and walked so many thousands of miles only to find myself at the highest weight I've ever been, one hundred and eighty four pounds. I'm only five foot three, so the look is not good. Clearly the diet and exercise strategy is a failure.

I've known for years that diets don't work. So why am I fat? Actually for the record I'm obese, so let's get that straight. I've been at this approximate weight for years now. I'm not gaining weight; I'm stable in that respect. The reason I'm fat is because my belief system has been totally compromised. But before we talk about solutions, let's take a look at the utter devastation that fat has brought to the entire world.

Chapter 2

The History of Fat

FAT HAS BEEN AROUND FOR A couple hundred years. I'm not talking about the naturally occurring fat that protects the body, but fat as an obsession, or social construct. Fat really came into its heyday sometime around the mid 1960's. I was a very little girl at the time, but I remember the world prior to the unleashing of fat. Back then people were naturally thin. No one went to the gym because there were no gyms. Hold on, okay that isn't entirely true. There were gyms, but basically their use was for amateur and professional boxers to do their training. I'm not kidding. In the real world Jack LaLanne was the only person doing a push-up. No one thought about fat at all. No one talked about fat. It just wasn't something to think about or talk about. It isn't that the topic of fat was taboo, fat as a topic simply did not exist. The only actual fat in our lives was on the side of a steak, and you could eat that if you enjoyed it. We ate butter and cheese. There was no rampant disease like we have today, and people actually died of something called "natural causes."

In the mid-sixties, society world-wide experienced quite the phenomenon. This was the advent of the first super-skinny supermodel, which arrived during the height of the 1960's British Invasion. Her name was Twiggy and she was naturally very thin. Don't get me wrong, I am not blaming Twiggy for a thing, I'm sure she's quite lovely. At the time anything coming out of London was the height of chic, so Twiggy got quite a bit of attention. It wasn't just the image of Twiggy that caused the problem, it was the exponential growth of the media, both television and print that pushed the problem along.

What happened was very interesting culturally. Women would look at Twiggy and instead of seeing her natural slenderness, they saw their own lack of thin by comparison, and fat was born. Not only was fat born, desperation to have an unnatural body was also born. Women wanted to look like Twiggy, and soon strategies to have the same body as her began cropping up.

Fat quickly became a problem, and when there's a problem, business and science become the solution. Sugar became the issue of focus and saccharine was invented. The business of fat is born. All soda brands began pushing out diet versions. By the early 1970's the first appetite suppressant came out called Aydds. They were little spongy chocolate-like squares in a box that actually looked like candy, and you were supposed to eat one if you felt hungry, thereby killing your appetite. Then diet pills, both prescription and over-the-counter began filling shelves. The diet books were being written by the dozen, and it became the language of the land to be on a diet. It wasn't whether you were on a diet or not, but rather which one. Being hungry was something that had to be stopped at all costs. Hunger went from nature's way to let you know your body is ready for nutrition, to something that needed to be eradicated. This was one of our first steps away from nature.

By the early 1980's sugar is still a villain, but our newest foe is fat grams. Manufacturers of processed food were making versions that were low fat and non-fat and good Lord in heaven the food was awful. Whole milk is totally off limits. Then down came the scourge of the universe, The Jane Fonda Workout Videos and books followed almost immediately by Richard Simmons. They were telling us if we don't work out we are going to get even fatter! Oh no! They put in a gym at my local YMCA, and Elaine Powers Fitness Clubs begin dotting the landscape. People start running and power walking. You have to get your cardio in! Yet we were getting fatter and fatter as each year rolls by. Fat becomes like alcoholism when Weight Watchers springs up and forces clients to be weighed in public. They must be accountable for their fat! They have meetings to talk about fat.

Suddenly there is disease devoted to fat. There is a steady and alarming increase in the cases of diabetes, heart disease and cancer. There are diseases invented in the fear of fat: Anorexia and Bullemia. The fear of fat becomes palpable throughout society. Suddenly carbs are bad and protein is good and we tell ourselves that as we step repeatedly on and off our stair stepper. And we get fatter and fatter until we get so fat that there needs to be a new word for how fat we are, and we come up with "obese." All the while we teach ourselves to hate what we've become.

Now, forty five years after The Fall of The Naturally Thin Empire, we find ourselves in The Culture of Fat.

Chapter 3

The Fat Cult

W HAT MAKES A GREAT CULT LEADER? Think about some of the greatest cult leaders known to man. Hitler was superb. Jim Jones did an outstanding job. Both of these gentlemen knew there were two ingredients keeping their followers in line. The first attribute is fear. A great cult leader knows if their followers fear them and fear what could happen to them if they defied their will, they could keep them in line. The second attribute is to program their minds into group think. If everyone thinks the same way then it has to be true, right? Go on, drink that Kool-Aid. Let's look at the dictionary meaning of the word cult and see if it doesn't fit like a glove. According to Dictionary.com: "Cult: Any system for treating human sickness that originated by a person usually claiming to have sole insight into the nature of the disease, and that employs methods regarded as unorthodox or unscientific."

Jack LaLanne was the first nutrition and exercise guru to hit the airwaves on television. He had credentials and was a Doctor of Chiropractic as well as a nutrition expert. He believed in fitness and good nutrition. These are all good things indeed. Somehow in the early 1980's his message of fitness and nutrition was bastardized by others correlating exercise with diet, weight loss and weight management. Jack LaLanne's message was skewed to the point of looking like it belonged in a house of mirrors. At the time the messages of weight loss, diet and exercise were coming at the public at warp speed, the public ended up buying it, and indulging in group think. Let's go to Dictionary. com for the definition of group think.

Group Think: the lack of individual creativity, or of a sense of personal responsibility, that is sometimes characteristic of group interactions.

Because we were being so bombarded by so called "experts" and "scientific study" we took in these messages in huge gulps, not taking the time to realize that the world never operated like this before.

Another way The Fat Cult gained popularity so quickly was feeding off of society's desperation to be unnaturally thin. Let's look at the Dictionary.com definition of despair and desperation:

Despair: loss of hope; hopelessness

Desperation: the state of being desperate or having the recklessness of despair

This makes perfect sense because when a mass of people are being assaulted with images of naturally thin bodies, and told this is how everyone should look, desperation for answers ensues. When one is desperate, according to the definition, they will act in reckless ways, and The Fat Cult fed directly off of this.

Remember, in 1965 society was naturally thin. In forty-five years we have literally gone collectively insane on the subject of fat. This is probably one of the biggest cases of group think in the history of humankind. We are cult members, and our cult leader's name is Fat. The cult captains are Diet and Exercise.

Chapter 4

The Language of Fat

THE LANGUAGE OF THE FAT CULT is one that is demeaning and unkind. When you look at the language of The Naturally Thin Empire, it was a fun place to be. We were thin or even skinny. We ate delicious food, and we played outside. We took leisurely walks, and we even strolled. Sporting a few extra pounds was just fine. "I'm pleasingly plump." "There's more of me to love."

The language of The Fat Cult is harsh and mean. Diet: Die-it. Exercise (work), Cardio (no fun), Lose (You're a Loser!); Weight (heavy); Weight Watchers (I'm watching my fat!); Belly Fat (horror!). We even have the television shows The Biggest Loser, My Six Hundred Pound Life, and Mike & Molly all focused on fat.

Back when I was a teen and perfectly naturally thin if someone walked up to me, got in my face and said "fuck you" I'd haul off and belt them in the mouth. Today teens greet each other with a rousing "fuck you" but God forbid one girl says to another "You're fat" and, well let's just say the eating disorder isn't far off. The word "fat" is used as a weapon to beat people down and to keep them in The Cult.

Chapter 5

The Insanity of Fat

REMEMBER, IN 1965 ZERO DOLLARS WERE spent on the business of fat. That's because there was zero market for the business. Why was there no market for the fat business, you ask? Because The Naturally Thin Empire was still holding power. Today, under The Fat Cult, the weight loss and exercise industry rakes in billions of dollars per year worldwide, and I haven't even begun to talk about the money medical industry pulls in. Yet we keep getting fatter. Of course there are people out there who legitimately have a metabolism issue, but I would imagine that they would be here on this earth at approximately the same percentage rate as 1965. But more than sixty percent of Americans are considered to be obese, and I would imagine that the percentage of obese Americans in 1965 was in the single digits, or less. Let us not forget there was a time when an obese woman's only job prospect was to be The Fat Lady in a circus side show. The rarity of obesity back then caused people to stop and stare in disbelief, and pay money for the opportunity. Today it is normal. What a mess we've made.

Now we have victims of fat looking for fat acceptance, and we have haters of fat people. You think the Republicans and Democrats are divided, look at fat and thin! We have boot camps for fat people and we have Jillian Michaels yelling at fat people on television. We have food addictions. We have good foods and bad foods. We get our stomachs stapled. We judge the content of our character based on our current waistline. We spend our precious time counting fat grams, carbs, repetitions, and hours exercising. We beat ourselves up emotionally, just to help our Cult Leader keep us in line. Then in our complete insanity we tithe money to The Cult in the form of membership dues, pre-packaged foods, supplements, cookbooks, magazines, all dedicated to fat. We pay fat to stay in the club. Then, when we actually get thin and the diet ends, we worry about fat, which makes us fat once again.

We worry about "good foods" and fear "bad foods." We all know what a good food is. A good food is broccoli and lettuce. Bad foods are pizza, hamburgers, hot dogs and cotton candy. In your wild insanity, ask yourself this. When you aren't dieting and you eat a piece of broccoli, do you beat yourself up for eating a good food while not dieting? There is no inherent goodness or badness in food. Food is what it is. Let's go to Dictionary.com:

Diet: A selection or a limitation on the amount a person eats for reducing weight (sounds pretty awful, huh?)

Eat: To take into the mouth and swallow for nourishment. To show enthusiasm for; take pleasure in (great!).

Let's take this total insanity one step further. The Fat Cult leaders have also programmed you with language inside of your own head to keep you in line. If you're pound abundant, think about the kinds of messages you say to yourself. I remember once I was at a Parent-Teacher Organization meeting, where at the time I was president. Naturally I had a lot of opportunities to speak in public. I have no problem with that, but I remember saying to myself before I took the stage: "You fat fuck, you don't deserve to be alive." If someone said that to one of my friends, or a family member I'd knock their block off, but I said this to myself and did it over and over again. I was verbally abusive to me. How steeped in sickness is that?

Chapter 6

Fat is a Liar

HERE ARE A FEW OF THE lies that fat tells us: The Freshman Fifteen; Fat runs in the family; Newlywed fat; It's hard to lose weight after you have a baby; It's hard to lose weight after the age of forty; It's hard to lose weight; You must diet and exercise to lose weight; You must deny yourself the foods you love to lose weight; You have to spend money to lose weight; If you're fat you're a loser; If you're fat you aren't as good as everyone else; You're a bad person; You have to do exercises you don't like to lose weight; Losing weight is hard work; Losing weight takes a long time; Fattening foods make you heavy. None of this is true.

Chapter 7

Your belief system and your body

WHAT YOU BELIEVE ABOUT YOUR BODY is your reality. Take a look at your body right now and it will scream at you what you believe. If you are overweight, you have any number of beliefs about food or exercise that are out of alignment with nature. If you are thin and perfect, you believe that you are thin and perfect and that is your reality. To prove this theory all I have to do is look at me. I eat very little food. I take in very little food and yet I'm fat. Calorically speaking, I really don't take in enough food to maintain my weight. If low calorie intake makes you thin, then I should be, by conventional reasoning, pencil thin, yet I'm not. Conversely, those with anorexia who can't see how desperately thin they are, continue to think thoughts of more thinness and this becomes their reality. You are the product of the thoughts you have thought about your body up to this moment. The good news is you can turn this around in an instant. You can align yourself with the truth of nature with the blink of an eye.

Chapter 8

Escape from the Cult

FIRST THINGS FIRST, QUIT THE CULT. I have been trying to get out of the Fat Cult for years now, but it keeps pulling me back in. Remember, the Cult is a liar and is insane. Look back on the previous chapters and see how you fit into the insanity. If you've never lived during The Naturally Thin Empire, seeing the insanity may be more difficult, but know that I am not lying to you about living in a naturally thin world. Also, you might take into consideration that there are no beer guts depicted in hieroglyphics or cave drawings. Indeed, there was once a world that spanned over the course of tens of thousands of years where natural thinness was the norm, and I'm ninety nine percent sure Jenny Craig had nothing to do with that. It's only in the last forty five years that we humans have really lost our minds. I'm going to break down the lies to you one by one:

- *The Freshman Fifteen:* So one time one kid gained fifteen pounds in his first semester away at college. Big flippin deal. Maybe he had a growth spurt.
- *Fat runs in the family:* There is no fat gene. If families tend to be fat it's because they are looking at each other's fat and they think about fat and they get fat.
- *Newlywed fat:* This is the weight you gain once the "I dos" are over and you can let down because you snagged your spouse. Baloney. If you expect you are going to gain weight right after the wedding, you most certainly will.
- *It's hard to lose weight after having a baby:* The chemical composition of fat cells is exactly the same before and after having a baby. It is easy to resume your natural state of thinness after having a baby.

- *It is hard to lose weight after the age of forty:* The chemical composition of fat cells is exactly the same before and after the age of forty. It is easy to resume your natural perfect weight after the age of forty.
- *It's hard to lose weight:* Indeed, but it is easy to resume your natural weight
- *You must diet and exercise to lose weight:* You may have to diet and exercise to lose weight, but you don't to restore your perfect body.
- *You must deny yourself foods that you love to lose weight:* True, but you can eat whatever you want while you resume your natural weight.
- *You need to spend money to lose weight:* Probably, but resuming your perfect skinny is always free of charge.
- *If you're fat you're a loser:* Your weight and your success as a human have nothing to do with one another
- *If you're fat you aren't as good as everyone else:* Adolph Hitler was slender.
- *You're a bad person:* Santa Claus seems like a good guy.
- *You have to do exercises you don't like to lose weight:* Yes, but you do not have to move your body at all to resume your natural weight
- *Losing weight is hard work.* Indeed, some of the hardest work I've ever done. Restoring my perfect weight is effortless.
- *Losing weight takes a long time:* Yup, sure does. Restoring your perfect body happens **very** quickly.
- *Fattening foods make you heavy:* There is no such thing as fattening food.
- *Feeling hunger is bad, you must stifle hunger:* Feeling hunger is good. It is nature's way of telling you you're ready for nutrition, and nourishment.
- *Eating food at night makes you fat:* Eating food is eating food, time of day does not matter
- *Losing more than one or two pounds per week is dangerous:* Really? What's going to happen am I going to get a hemorrhoid?

Chapter 9

The Struggle

I HEAR PEOPLE SAY IT ALL the time, and I'm guilty of saying the same thing. "I'm struggling with my weight," or "I have struggled with my weight all of my life." Let's go back to Dictionary.com.

"Struggle: To contend with an adversary or opposing force."

According to the Law of Attraction, you attract what it is you're fighting. Back in 1965 we were not fighting fat, therefore we weren't attracting it. This is why these so called "wars" we keep waging keep making matters worse. There is the War on Drugs. More people are addicted to drugs than before the war started. There's the fight against breast cancer, and there is more breast cancer now than ever. Fighting attracts more of what you don't want in your life.

So to say you're struggling with your weight means you are in an unending fight with your own body. This is true in my case. The minute I believed the first myth forty years ago, I literally declared war on my body. I believed the newlywed myth, then the baby myth, and so on. I have been at war with my body for forty years. It's time for a truce.

Chapter 10

How to get started

THE FIRST THING YOU NEED TO do is to deprogram yourself from The Cult. Accept your body the way it is now. Go into peace talks with yourself. End the struggle. If you don't do that you will keep beating yourself up which will hold back the great result you are looking for. Remember, the way your body looks today is the direct response to the thoughts you have thought in the past. Beginning now, and we don't have to wait until Monday with this plan, you will replace any negative fat thoughts with a positive thin thought. So let's say you're driving in your car and you hit a pot hole and you notice your six-pack abs jiggle a little. Laugh and say "it is what it is." Your affirmation should be something like *I am beautiful the way I am and I will still be beautiful when I arrive at my perfect weight.* This will get you started today, and it's the truth.

Now, one of the most important things you will need to do for yourself is to get to know and like you. If you aren't at your perfect weight right now, chances are you have been pretty mean to yourself. Remember me telling myself I was a fat fuck? That hurt. Think about the person inside of you, your being, your spirit. The part of you that goes on when you shed the meat suit. That person doesn't have a weight issue. Be kind to that person and treat him/her with love. Learn to love yourself and you will never send another negative message again.

What I really want you to do is fall in love with you. It's amazing to me how easy it was to become my own abuser. We need to turn that around and fall head over heels in love with ourselves. Remember that feeling the first time you fell in love with another? When you fell in love with another, you attracted a wonderful person into your life that made your life so much better. Imagine what amazing things you will bring

17

to yourself if you feel that way about you. When you fall in love with yourself you see yourself completely honestly for the first time in your life. You see what others see in you. Change the conversation in your mind from one of ugliness to one of nurturing.

Use your emotions as your guide. You can't think about what you think about all day long. Frankly it would be exhausting, and you probably wouldn't get much done. Understand that your only job in this life is to live like my dog Lily. Be happy with spikes of joy. Know that, whenever you feel a negative emotion, especially in reference to your body, change it immediately to a positive emotion, or even a neutral one. It just might be one of those old harsh criticisms you had a habit of leveling on yourself. It might be The Cult trying to lure you back in. It may take some time to change that habit, but it is well worth changing. Some may think that you're lying to yourself with these positive affirmations, but honestly, fake it until you make it. You will see things happen.

Chapter 11

Get Clear on What You Want

IN ORDER TO RESTORE YOUR PERFECT natural weight, all you have to do is set your sights on what it is you want. When you get clear on what it is you want, be very careful to make sure you don't ask for what you don't want. For instance, if you think "I don't want to be fat," that is still a fat thought, and that's what you'll get. Instead, think about restoring your perfect thinness. Identify a time in your adult/teen life when you were at your perfect thinness. For me it was when I was one hundred and eighteen pounds. If you've never been at your perfect thinness, pick a weight that seems believable for you. Ignore height/ weight charts. That applies the same standard to everyone, which is not realistic. Everyone is different and their perfect thinness can and does vary widely.

Once you have identified the weight that you wish to be, you now have vision. You can see yourself at this weight. Maybe you have pictures of yourself at this weight, so you know with absolute certainty that it is possible for you to be at this weight because you have been there before effortlessly

A powerful way to bring what you want to you more quickly is to visualize. There are many ways to exercise visualization techniques. Right now I have a vision board on my refrigerator that has a picture of a woman with the most amazing body, and perfect rock solid abs. I look at that picture every single day and visualize myself looking like that. Meditation is another way to get visualizing going. Get into a quiet place and relax your entire body. When your body is totally relaxed, begin concentrating on your breathing. Listen to your breathing and slow it down a little bit. Once you are in a state of complete relaxation begin visualizing your body as you imagine it will look. Imagine your body parts getting smaller and smaller. This will powerfully pull your perfect body to you even faster.

Chapter 12

Eat and be Joyful!

Now listen to this....I'm actually telling you that exercise is not necessary, but then recommend that you exercise. Don't listen to me; I'm still in The Cult!

YOU KNOW THOSE ANNOYING SKINNY PEOPLE who say "I eat whatever I want and I'm always thin"? Honestly, do you know the difference between them and us? One teensy weensy little thing. They absolutely one hundred percent believe the statement they made. I once had a co-worker that was like this. She not only ate what society would call "fattening" foods, she ate them in absolute abundance. She believed that she was a thin person, and that she could eat whatever she wanted, and this was her truth. This can become our truth as well. But we honestly have to believe it. If you are currently not at your perfect weight like me, you have belief systems that are out of tune with nature, just like me.

Back when I was a kid, and even into my teen years, I ate whatever I wanted. The goodness or badness of food was based solely on flavor. My mother cooked with butter and put butter on vegetables to get us to eat them. We were all thin as rails. My mother cooked with bacon grease. My mother would melt a couple tablespoons of bacon grease and put it into homemade cole slaw. It was unbelievably good and we were thin as rails. She made pie crust using lard and we were thin as rails.

Eat what you like. No food is off limits if you like it. If you feel like having pizza, have pizza. If you don't like spinach, don't eat it. Take the goodness and badness out of food. Food is just food. There are regular and low fat versions of just about all foods. Eat the version you enjoy the most. For instance with saltine crackers, in the brand I buy, I happen to like the fat free version better because it's crunchier than the original version. As long as you are making your food choices out of preference, and not out of lack of calories you are making an excellent choice. I know people who are not dieting and they enjoy the taste of diet soda over the original.

When it comes to exercise this is completely up to you. Back in the 1960's my mother did not exercise a lick. She didn't go on walks, go swimming or anything. She was five feet tall and one hundred and two pounds, which was a perfect weight for her frame. For the sake of the integrity of the theories I am positing here I will not deliberately exercise so that I can prove to you that this can be done, and done easily. However, that doesn't mean that I'm not going to move my body. That doesn't mean that I'm not going to take my dogs for walks. I like doing that. But please, only move your body in ways you like. Let me tell you why.

The last time I lost weight I didn't diet because even five years ago I knew diets don't work. I was in graduate school so I was home during the day. In the morning I would walk with one dog for an hour, and in the afternoon I would walk the other for another hour, because this is something I enjoy, although I was actively trying to lose weight. In between the walks I did an exercise DVD to work my abdominals, a perceived problem area. Well I really had a mixed result. My overall body was about a size six, but my abdominals were a size eight. I had to wear baggy size eight clothes to accommodate my abdominals. I hated doing the DVD and it showed. I would have been better off not doing the DVD at all and I would have had size six all over.

I have a sister-in-law that loves to workout at the gym, and it shows. She has a beautiful figure because she loves what she does. If you do something you don't like you will definitely have a poor result. Consider it play rather than working out. Some of the happiest people I know play for exercise. Get out your video game console and play some tennis, or one of those dancing games, or hit those free weights hard if that's what you like. Go for a bike ride, but do it because you feel like having fun, rather than a chore that you must complete. If the way you move your body is a chore, simply don't do it. Pick something else.

You may be asking yourself why I gained the weight back and then some after the last attempt five years ago? Those old familiar lies came back into play. I went back to school full time, and perceived that the only reason I lost the weight in the first place was because of the walking, and I knew I was not going to have the time, so the weight was going to come back on, and it did. The reason I lost the weight was NOT because I was walking, but because I BELIEVED I was losing weight. When my thoughts changed to the negative, absolutely knowing that I was going to gain the weight that became my reality.

One of the tricks I use to keep the skinny thoughts in the forefront of my mind is to limit the amount of media I'm exposed to. I don't listen to the radio in the car. There are too many commercials for weight loss products and diets. I record the television shows I like to watch so I can fast forward through the commercials. I know advertisers don't want to hear this, but the weight loss and diet industries are really negative, but then again they are the Masters of the Cult. I mean there is one commercial out there that shows this person with huge belly fat, and the opening line is "Belly fat make you angry?" Hell, I don't want to look at belly fat and I don't want to be angry! The commercial should say "Perfect abs make you happy!"

Finally, stop looking at labels. You don't need to count calories, fat grams or carbs. In fact so many packaged items come into my home with the words "Fat free" or "low fat" that I made up labels that say "slender abundant" and I cover up the offending swear word. We just don't do the "F" word in my house anymore.

Today is Thursday, June 3, 2010. I weigh one hundred and eighty four pounds. Beginning today I am going to allow my body to return to its normal natural weight. In the pages that follow will be the journal I keep in order for you to follow my progress. Wish me luck!

January 25, 2011

Hello readers, it's me Laura. This is the part of the book where I begin journaling. It had been a long time since I had written the first twelve chapters. Read on...

That was seven months ago, and for the most part I stand by what I've written. Have I resumed my perfect weight yet? The answer to that would be a rousing no. Getting out of the cult is more difficult than I thought. When I wrote what I did in the preceding pages, I understood it intellectually. What I failed to factor in is the emotional hold the Fat Cult has over me. I have been a hostage of the Fat Cult. I am behaving like a hostage. There is a very real part of me that continues to try to please my oppressors, and over the last seven months I have tithed to them repeatedly. I bought a treadmill. I bought weights. I bought a body building machine. I probably spent close to two thousand dollars. As Bugs Bunny would say, "What a maroon!" I know what I know intellectually, but emotionally I am still dependent on The Cult to keep me in line.

There are a few things I would like to concede to. First, as humans, it is really good for us to move our bodies. Our bodies were designed to move. You simply can't be a nomad or a hunter/gatherer without moving your body. Also, moving your body feels good. Moving your body doesn't have to be painful, in fact it shouldn't be painful at all. Moving your body should be pleasant and fun. Moving your body is part of our overall good health. It strengthens bones, and the heart. It is a catalyst for excellent health. Bottom line? Moving your body is great for you.

Some may argue that with technology we are more sedentary than ever. This is true, but it doesn't have to be true. In my old job, during the course of my day, the cubicle would often feel like it was closing in on me, and I'd get up and take a couple laps around the office. Last week I replaced my office chair, here in my trusty office with an exercise ball. I prefer to call it a "bouncy ball" because I'm having fun. I get to bounce and stretch while I'm writing, which is floating my boat.

I will defend my treadmill purchase. I love to walk, but I live in a climate where walking outdoors, which I prefer, is only really reasonable to do from April through October. Having a treadmill takes weather out of the equation. I can walk whenever I want to. I also love walking with my mp3 player, and I end up dance walking, which is way fun. I really love that. It just doesn't feel like exercise when I'm doing something I love.

It's funny but I'm thinking back to when I was a kid. I realize that my experience as a kid was different than a lot of kids now. When we got home from school, we'd have a snack. In the good weather my mother and pretty much all mothers back then, forced their kids out the door and said "go play." It was an innocent time. Kids didn't have play dates; they just showed up and played. In my neighborhood we rode bikes in packs, jumped in leaves, played "Red light, green light" or "Mother may I" which I think may be the same game. We played hopscotch and four squares, and we went home for dinner when the street lights came on. Like I said, it was an innocent time. The activities we involved ourselves in we never considered exercise. It was just play. When I was a teenager, I didn't play hopscotch anymore, but I routinely had dance parties in my room to some very loud music. I moved my body and I felt good all of the time. None of this was a chore; in fact it was a pleasure, pure pleasure.

Today, knowing I was going to start fresh with a new attitude, I looked over what games I have for my video game console. I have fitness video game that calculates my weight and calories burned. Kill me. The Spouse gave me Jillian Michaels Fitness Ultimatum for Christmas. The wrapper isn't even off. Fitness Ultimatum, can you think of anything less inspiring? I mean, I'm sorry Jillian. You have the best intentions in the world, but really, Fitness Ultimatum? When was the last time someone gave you an ultimatum that was positive? Try this on: Eat this cupcake or I might just be forced to give you a kiss! It doesn't work. An ultimatum is always negative, always. The Fitness Ultimatum: Do this or be fucking fat. There you go.

So, what is my game plan here? First, I need to feel good about me. I am pretty awesome. I realize that the state my body is currently in, is simply a result of the thoughts I have thought, up until now. Today the new thoughts begin. I am a thin person. My goal is to have fun every day. When I come home from work, I will put on my play clothes and play. My entire aim is to have a great time and play to my heart's content. I will continue making delicious and balanced meals for myself and my family, and enjoy those fun meals like pizza and fast food in moderation. I will stop exercising and start playing. Beginning today I will go on a nice walk after dinner each night. In the good weather I will walk with my dogs, and in the poor weather I will walk on my treadmill. I love walking. It makes me happy. I will play with my video games every day and have fun. I will resume my perfect weight by May. I am so excited about this. What a great time to be me! I am so happy!

January 28, 2011

It's time we talked about numbers. I knew I never liked math for a reason. The reason is numbers. Are numbers useful? Yeah, maybe for some things like preheating the oven, or measuring wood, or calculating missile codes, or other stuff like that, but I'm finding out more and more that numbers are as misleading and subjective as words. At least the way we humans interpret them. Let's take a look at numbers, and how we perceive our bodies, and how it has worked out for us.

One of the first things that come to mind is how I punish myself over my weight and what size I am. If I'm a size six, I'm good, but if I'm a sixteen, it's bad. Size is just a number, and while we may want to use it as a measuring stick, I think we need to rethink that. We can't let our size, good or bad determine our happiness, and we do, but it just isn't worth it. Size is another captain in the Fat Cult. If dress size were uniform and standardized, I might just acquiesce a little bit on it because then it could be argued that size is something that has been agreed upon. So a size eight would always be a size eight, no matter what designer, or what country the garment was made in. However this isn't the case. Size is totally up to the manufacturer. I can be a sixteen in one brand and a twelve in another. I have a name brand jacket that I bought at a big box club store that is a XXXL. I guarantee that the manufacturer of said garment sold the jackets in bulk to this store because the sizes were mislabeled. The point is, I bought the jacket in XXXL because the jacket fit, not the size. So let's throw dress size to the wind. We simply cannot aspire to a dress size because you can't aspire to something that doesn't exist. Thank God, that was a huge burden.

Let's take a look at the required nutritional label on food. Stop looking at it. There are so many things that people are fixating on with that label, it is downright sinful. Fat grams, calories, carb grams, protein grams, salt. Let it go. If you want it, have it. Stop counting everything in sight. It's almost like we've become an OCD society, and all we do is count things when it comes to food. Good Lord, it takes all the pleasure out of eating. Eat in moderation, and if you don't know what moderation is, consult with a nutritionist, or look online, eat slowly, and listen for your body to tell you you're full. Spend the time you would be spending counting calories and logging them on Weight Watchers.com on enjoying time with your family. Counting calories, and the related cousins of fat, protein and carbs have only done one thing: Made us fat.

Last on the counting list; stop counting how much time you put into exercising. If you're goal is to have fun, then why are you counting? When you were a little kid, did you say "hmmm I'm going to have one hour of fun, and then I have to stop and do something unfun for a while." No, you had fun for as long as you wanted and as long as it remained fun. Fun isn't something you put time constraints on. So if you enjoy walking on your treadmill like me, don't worry about the time, just have fun. Don't put it on your "to do" list because you only put unfun things on the to-do list, not fun things. I don't need to be reminded to have fun. I have fun. I need to be reminded to clean the litter box or take out the trash, but going to the beach just doesn't need to be on the to-do list. Stop turning an opportunity for fun into a chore. The Fat Cult already did that for you.

March 3, 2011

Hi, it's me. Don't do what I talk about here.

I can feel myself well on the way to my perfect body now. I feel my abdominals strengthening and slimming. Up until today I've been going on the exercise ball, and putting my feet on my treadmill, and working my abs to the music, which I like well enough. I like moving my body that way. But it is only okay. My results have been fair so far, but today I think I really discovered what it is I enjoy a lot ....I like dancing on the exercise ball. You need to know that I really like the exercise ball. When I commandeered this space and made it into my office a few months ago, I got rid of the horrible office chair that was in here, and rather than replacing it with yet another chair, I just put an exercise ball in its place.

Today I started dancing on my exercise ball. Hold it right there. I hate the term "exercise ball." I've seen it called a "Fitness Orb" which nearly made me pee my pants. Let's see, what could we call it? Hmmmmm. I think I am going to call it what it is. It's a bouncy ball. For the record, this is how you dance on a bouncy ball. Sit in the middle of the ball, with your feet planted firmly on the floor. I suggest you wear sneakers, or your feet could come out from under you and you'll hit the deck. Put on your mp3, or your WalkMan or Boom Box or Victrola and pick music that you like and start bouncing and dancing. The great thing about this is no one is telling you how to do it, or what music you have to listen to. It is all your choice. It's like my old dance parties from when I was a teenager, only with a bouncy ball. I'm going to call this a bouncy ball dance party. Now I'm not saying you need to do this. Do what you like to do. If you like to jump rope, jump rope. If you like to hop on a pogo stick, do that. If you are morbidly obese, you can begin moving too. Do what I do while sitting on your couch. Put on your headset or stereo and have a dance party. Move your arms and feet like you are dancing and imagine your perfect body while you're doing it. Before long you will feel your body begin to change, and you will begin transforming yourself into the you you are meant to be.

One of the things I've learned along the way, during this journey of discovery about how nature works, is that when you feel the need to control something, you are working against the very thing you desire. Think about all the things we seek to control in our world. Gun control...more guns now than ever before. Disease control....more disease than ever before. Weight control....more obesity than ever before. Let's go back to dictionary.com:

"Control: to exercise restraint or direction over; dominate; command."

So here we go again. Control is a struggle, and if we are struggling we are moving away from the very thing we desire. Have you ever seen anyone try to control a child at the mall who wants to go into the toy store? I don't know about you but it usually doesn't work out well for the grown-ups.

One of the things I wanted to talk about is our clothes. How we suffer over clothes. Those of us who have carried extra weight over the years really batter ourselves. We are told over and over, not to buy ourselves anything in the size we are currently in, but rather in a smaller size so that when we lose the weight we will look so cute. Let me clue you in on something. When we lose the weight we will look really cute whether we have the smaller clothes or not. The problem with running your wardrobe this way is that eventually you will have a closet full of clothes that don't fit, and nothing in the right size. This has happened to me, and it is the state of my closet currently. So now I'm depressed over not fitting into the clothes that were supposed to be the carrot that got me to lose the weight, AND I have nothing in the closet that makes me feel good now.

Our only responsibility on this earth and in our lifetime is to be happy. If we are anything but happy, we are simply not doing our job. To look into a closet full of clothes that are too small, and to feel bad about what we are wearing is sheer insanity. In what parallel universe does one go to a department store and deliberately purchase a clothing item that does not fit, and then walk around wearing rags. This is stupid personified, and yet I have done this over and over for years.

Because we are supposed to be happy, and we are supposed to love ourselves, that type of behavior should be off limits. If you love yourself, you love yourself no matter what size you are. You are beautiful and you deserve to look beautiful no matter what size you are. Never deprive yourself of beautiful things. Wearing beautiful clothes in the right size, no matter what that size is, is going to make you feel one hundred times better than having a closet full of clothes that are too small, and rags to wear in public. I can't believe I did this to myself, and I sure hope I can stop you from doing it to yourself anymore. It is yet another Cult Classic lie.

Save those purchases for when you actually do fit into that size, and then imagine how it will feel to buy the smaller size, and actually try it on in the changing room. Imagine trying that item on, and having it fit, and buying it and wearing it out in public. How fun is that?

Resuming our perfect weight, is much different that losing weight, or gaining skinny. Resuming our perfect weight simply means defaulting to factory settings. When you set your computer or mp3 player to its default settings, all it does is wipe out whatever you've put into the device, and return it to the state it was in when you took it out of the box. This isn't to say that you will become eight pounds six ounces, like at birth. When I say "factory settings" I mean the ideal weight you were meant to weigh before you fell for the myths and stopped deliciously moving your body. To lose weight is to constantly be on the cycle of gaining and losing and honestly isn't that something we've already done probably ten to fifteen times in our lifetime? Gaining skinny, which sounds much more positive, is equally a hamster wheel. If you need to gain your skinny, it means you lost your skinny too. Round and round and round we go. Resuming your perfect weight and defaulting to factory settings is the way to never have to worry about it ever again. Once we resume our perfect weight, and learn to move our bodies the way nature wants us to for health and vitality, we will jump off the hamster wheel for good.

While we're in pursuit of our factory settings, I want you to think about the clothes you are currently wearing. Our clothes are sort of like our daily version of The Three Bears story. Clothes can be too big, too small, or just right. Just like I suggested that you not to buy clothes that are too small, I am also suggesting you don't wear clothes that are too small. If you're a size twelve and you are squeezing yourself into a size ten pants, you are not going to feel like you're wearing a size ten. You'll feel like you're a size sixteen, and you'll look like ten pounds of garbage forced into a five pound bag. Only wear clothes that make you feel good. If you have that pair of slacks that squeezes your love handles, don't wear them. All you will think about all day long are your love handles, and if you're thinking about love handles, you are getting love handles. What I do is try to wear clothes that are a little bit too big. When my clothes don't squeeze me in places that make me feel uncomfortable, I automatically feel thin. The more often you feel thin during the day, the more often you think thin, and when you think thin, you attract thin, and when you attract thin, you become thin. You want a really great tip for feeling and thinking thin for nearly half your day? Wear pajamas a size too big. I don't know about you, but I'm in my jammies nearly half my day. If you can feel thin half your day, imagine how quickly you will begin attracting it to you.

Before I close for the day, one of the things I want to address is food. Food gets such a bad rap. It's really a shame because food is awesome. First things first, if you have a psychological or emotional reason, or you think you might, for eating the amount of food you eat, you will want to go to a counselor or psychologist to eliminate those issues before, or while, we go on this amazing adventure. If you have been victimized in your life, and you think it is possible that you cope with your situation using food, then this is something that I can't help you with, but will be here to help you once you put to rest that awful thing that has caused this. I'm patient. I will be right here.

For the rest of us who have not been traumatized, the fix is really simple, anything in moderation. I simply have one helping of my meal, and that's it. Somehow as a people, we have gone from feeling satisfied and sated after a meal, to needing to feel stuffed to the gills. Growing up, we only did that once a year and that was at Thanksgiving. Thanksgiving was the only holiday during the year that was all about the consumption of food. Heck, you couldn't even get a turkey at the grocery store any other time of year. Turkey was such a rare treat that we ate ourselves into a coma once a year.

You can eat whatever you want as long as it's in moderation. If you need to relearn what a healthy portion of food is, then there are nutritionists, dieticians, and all sorts of resources on the Internet to help you identify what a healthy portion is. Now, don't get me wrong, I'm not talking about portion control....that would be a bad thing. The minute we go into "portion control" the struggle over what is enough and what isn't enough begins again, and the scales come out, and we start counting points, and we weigh ourselves in public....OH God! Look at pictures of healthy portions and learn how to eyeball. For me, a perfect portion means that I have meat, vegetable, starch (rice, pasta, potato), and maybe a piece of bread or biscuit (mmmmm biscuits) on my plate with space in between them. You can also use butter on your biscuit. Have a bowl of soup and some bread. Enjoy a bowl of pasta and some bread (cheese too!). Savor a nice bowl of cereal. Eat whatever you want in moderation.

There are two ends of the food consumption continuum. On one end is deprivation. We deny ourselves food we enjoy in the misguided quest to be thin. Then when this becomes too painful, and it does become too painful for most, the trip to the other end of the line is all too quick and easy: Gluttony. Eating everything that isn't nailed down. Gluttony is equally as disastrous as deprivation. Equally as painful, and it becomes the vicious cycle that we now call diet and exercise. Let us go back to the beginning. Our job on this earth is to be happy. What is it about this scenario that makes us happy? Nothing, absolutely nothing. There is no joy.

We are supposed to be happy with spikes of joy. We are supposed to live a life full of abundance. We are supposed to enjoy the sensuous nature of food. Food is to be savored. It is no mistake that often when we have an off-the-charts gastronomic experience, the sounds that emanate from our bodies are extremely similar to sexual satisfaction noises. I call a moment like that a FoodGasm. When you participate in a particularly satisfying sexual experience, it is better when the peak is reached slowly and with great care and attention to detail. This makes the orgasm unique, spine tingling, and toe curling. When we engage in gluttony, we've stuffed ourselves so quickly, we haven't taken the time to savor and enjoy. The meal is over with a burp and a fart. This is the gastronomic version of premature ejaculation.

April 2, 2011

So today I decided that I really deserve to have clothes that fit. I went shopping and got some spring clothes, but when I got them home and tried them on (too permanently traumatized by dressing rooms to do it in the store) they were too small. I debated bringing them back, but they are spring clothes, and we're still a few weeks away from actually being able to wear them, so I think I'll keep them. By the time the weather is right to wear them, I'll be in that size, and so it works out. However I went to a fancy department store and bought two pairs of jeans that I really want to wear beginning now. They too were too small. I'm going to return them. I'm not keeping what isn't right for me.

I think the best way to approach this is to say that I'm a size 7JA06-77Z and call it a day. I refuse to let the clothes I bought today get me down. Right now I'm going to go online to find jeans that fit and order them right away.

I really am a moron. I kept the spring clothes that don't fit and returned the jeans. I never did order new jeans.

April 5, 2011

In this chapter you will see how I manage to keep getting sucked back into The Cult even though intellectually I understand these concepts.

I guess I have to admit that I did let it get me down. I am still struggling with The Cult to get out. I am absolutely permanently traumatized by changing rooms at the mall, and I'd rather buy something and return it than to go in there again. NEVER! Anyway, I managed to really make myself feel bad because some of the clothes didn't fit. I ended up following my own advice and returning the jeans that didn't fit. The other clothes that I got are spring clothes, and we are still struggling with cold weather here in the great Garden State, so I decided to keep them in anticipation of being able to wear them in a couple months when it is really warm. If I can't wear them for some reason....if I've really failed miserably, I will document that too. I am laying myself naked here. You are getting the Laura that only my family sees. So hopefully all of those designer clothes I bought will be happily draped on my body shortly....even though I don't believe in this stupid practice. Oh Grrrrr to me!

When did we lose our sense of fun? When was it beaten out of us? I remember looking forward to certain dinners my mother would make when I was a kid because I loved it so much. I would "save my appetite," a concept largely lost, and wait for this terrific dinner. Today it seems that along with looking forward to a fabulous meal, we are also anticipating what price we are going to pay for it the next day. Again, there will be numbers associated with the meal. We will gain five pounds, or maybe we will have to run that extra mile to take it off. When we obsess about anything, by definition we have stripped the joy out of that which we are obsessing. Obsessing is rooted in anxiety. You don't need to be a licensed psychotherapist to know this. Simply look up the definition. If we are obsessing, we cannot enjoy anything. We have stripped the joy.

The gain and loss of weight is completely between our ears. Let me give you an example from my life. Back when my daughter was a baby, we were poor and only had one car. My husband needed the car to go to work, so I was stuck without. The baby stroller became my car. Every day my daughter and I would walk everywhere we needed to go. I kept telling myself that I was going to have the most gorgeous beautiful body ever because of this, and guess what? I did! But when we weren't so poor and I got my own car and I started driving everywhere, I knew I would gain the weight back because now I was driving instead of walking, and sure enough the weight came back. Now conventional scientific wisdom would say, sure, you stopped walking and of course the weight came back. Back when I was a teenager I walked everywhere and was perfectly slim. You may take that statement to support what happened above. But then I got my first car when I was seventeen years old, and guess what. I drove everywhere and didn't gain an ounce....until I bought the newlywed myth. All weight gain and loss is due to what our current belief system is between our ears.

I'm expecting all sorts of criticism from lots of different people. I fully expect the diet and exercise industry to come unglued over what I'm saying. I'm expecting the medical industry to take me to task. The most difficult group I will have to encounter is the younger people.... born after 1980, who never saw a world that wasn't obese. People who never experienced a world where there was peace on this topic. Worse yet, young doctors who may have never seen for themselves, a perfectly thin world, and are steeped in the research and medicine of fat. They might be the toughest group of all. But the fact of the matter is things haven't always been this way. The human body has not morphed. I mean if the human body was to morph in some way, according to the Law of Natural Selection, it is going to evolve in a way that causes it to become healthier, and to adapt to its environment. This is certainly not the case. Fat is not in our genes. Having sixty percent of our society considered obese is not evolution. To evolve is to produce an even better and more refined version than the iteration before. We are devolving. There is a reason for this. We believe all the wrong things. Then we promote these beliefs, and study them, and research them, and scientifically document them, and micromanage them until, because some of this is based in science, we actually believe it, because, heck, it's science, right? Wrong.

What has happened is we believe all the wrong things. We've bought into the notion that we have to control our weight, when in reality, we do not. It will take care of itself, but we have to change our thinking. It has taken me time to shed the beliefs I have, and honestly I'm still working on it. I have been programmed like you. The tethers of belief of what I've been told about my body and fat for the last forty years run extremely deep, and I often find that I'm shocked when I indulge one of them.

Letting go of those beliefs is much more difficult than you think. The Cult has many more resources than we do to keep us around, and to keep us convinced that they are right and our nature is wrong, many more. Think about it. The media, who I believe is the Marketing Director of The Cult, is right on the front line. You can't turn on the television or radio without being assaulted by commercials for weight loss products, gym memberships, pills, surgery, low fat food, and all sorts of other scare tactics. Remember, one of the most effective forms of advertising is to scare the crap out of you. That's why we are bad breath fearing germaphobes.

I will confess that I've been in a fairly media free life for a long time. I don't listen to the radio in my car, and mostly I record the TV shows I like to watch on my DVR so I can fast forward through the commercials. When my husband is home and we watch TV together he tends to surf during the commercials, so I don't see them. This is one defense. Another is to select the magazines I read carefully. I don't waste my time on garbage, and only subscribe to magazines that make me feel good about me. You may say that it isn't healthy not knowing what is going on in the world. Ha! Try to not know. If there is something I need to know, I find out about it. The cost of constant engagement in the world is way too high sometimes.

One of the things I keep haranguing about in this book, is that it is our job on this earth to be loving and happy. That's it, loving and happy. Yet, the miserable wretches that we are, we do the exact opposite. We are miserable most of the time. I look the people who pass through my life and I'm amazed at how they get through their day sometimes. They begin so many sentences with "I'm so annoyed" or "I'm so irritated."

Yeah, that's a happy life! I look at my dogs Lily and Riley and those are happy and loving beings. You know what? Let's explore Lily and Riley's lives a little bit. Let's see what we can learn from them.

First off, I do believe my dogs have a sense of fun. All I have to do is take out the dog leash and Lily is quite literally jumping off the ground ready to lose her mind. I don't think she's thinking "Oh crap that leash again....I guess we have to go for a walk...damn it." No! She can't get out of the door fast enough. When we get going on our walk, she walks with great purpose, with her head up, and a great big grin on her face. Some of you who aren't dog lovers will argue that the dog simply does not smile. Well you're wrong, she does smile, and people who see her on her walk, inevitably stop me and want to visit with her because she is in such a state of absolute joy. When I take Riley, he is equally as joyful, but expresses a little differently. He wants to enjoy every odor he can find on the walk. He too smiles a great big contented smile the entire time we walk. They would walk all day every day if I had the time. Walking isn't exercise to them, its love. It's joy.

Let's talk about my dogs and food. Every day I put out the same food in the same bowl. There has never been a time when either of my dogs have looked at the bowl and looked at me and said "Dude, Really? Again?" No, they happily eat their food whenever they feel hungry, and then stop when they've had enough. Did you just hear what I said? They eat their food whenever they feel hungry, and then stop when they've had enough. I have yet to see any of my dogs eat to the point of gluttony, unzip their pants and say "I was full, but I kept eating because it is sooooo good!"

Here is the bottom line. My dogs, whose brains have far less computing power than our human brains, have managed to strike a balance that eludes us humans when it comes to food. My dogs live to be happy and loving. Walking with me makes them happy. Playing stick in the yard makes them happy. Sitting on the front porch with me, makes them happy. Eating a bowl of dog food makes them happy. Having the occasional cat treat makes them happy. You may argue that they are far less complex than we are. True. But we can learn a whole lot about simplifying our lives through them.

I've been spending some time looking online for a mental disorder that I could label what it is we do when we continue on the hamster wheel of diet and exercise. It seems to me that society is suffering from an anxiety based social phobia which gets reinforced over and over so that our brains are tricked into believing what is a lie. This is what The Cult does. The Cult has created a widespread social phobia that never existed before, and like a good bureaucracy, this phobia lives to make sure it continues living no matter what. In the face of all other evidence to the contrary, this man-made, media-supported phobia not only remains strong, it grows exponentially. Without putting a stop to it, will 70% of American's be obese in 2012? The Cult has become a self-fulfilling prophecy that is "this close" to having its own diagnostic codes. I propose to name what we are suffering from Social Weight Anxiety Disorder (SWAD). Let's look at the symptoms of SWAD:

- The obsessive need to go on and off a diet
- The obsessive need to begin aggressive exercise plans
- Mondays are always the start date. The weekend before is used to gain more weight to take off
- Performing exercises that are unpleasant, and at times of the day that are not fun
- Eating foods which are unpleasant or unsatisfying, or both
- Constant worry about weight, and comparing weight with others
- Dislike of oneself, due to body image
- Destructive internal dialog with self
- Seeking confirmation from others that one isn't/is fat
- Scrutinizing foods for their goodness or badness of calories or fat
- Obsessively keeping record of calories consumed, exercises performed, fat grams consumed.
- Defining success by the scale, or by an "expert" who determines what they should weigh

- When the diet either ends or the dieter "blows it" the emotional pounding that takes place when "bad" food is reintroduced
- The anxiety and heartbreak when weight comes back on when the diet ends.

I can't believe that there isn't anyone out there other than me who thinks that there needs to be a diagnosis for what society is going through. The reason I believe there needs to be a diagnosis is because THIS ISN'T NORMAL! This isn't right. These symptoms were never experienced prior to the mid 1960's. This is man-made, and not something nature would produce.

If being at a perfect normal healthy weight is being in a state of ease, then being overweight or obese is being in a state of dis-ease and that dis-ease needs a name. We call it overweight. We call it obesity. Okay, sure fine. That's what it is, but it doesn't explain why. Once we understand the why, we can treat it, and bring our society back to its default normal. It may take several lifetimes to do this, but we have to start somewhere, and the time is now.

One of the things I have come to understand is that, for the most part, we humans are seriously disconnected from nature. We are disturbed to find out that the meat we eat is farmed, and that the animals are deliberately slaughtered for our consumption. For so many of us, we are completely disconnected even from our own back yards. We pay landscapers to take care of our property, and we largely live our lives inside of our hermetically sealed homes. We are also grossly disconnected from our bodies as well. Because we are either stuffing our bodies with food, or denying ourselves nutrition, in either event this is totally against nature. Our bodies are born with a natural rhythm to it. This is why babies cry when they're hungry.

When my daughter was born, my pediatrician told me to never feed her more than once in two hours. Being a rule follower myself, I did adhere to this rule, until I realized that I was fighting nature, and my kid. Her body rhythm wanted her to feed every hour and a half, three times in a row, followed by a solid eight hours of sleep. My baby was trying like the dickens to be awake during the day and sleep at night, but because I bought into this whole control thing I was fighting what was her nature. When I finally gave in and fed according to her needs, the struggle stopped and she was a happy baby. I learned quickly that asking a newborn baby to wait a half hour to eat involves a lot of crying and screaming and the baby hates it too.

When my son was born, he grew like you can't believe. By the time he was eight months old, he was twenty four pounds. He was as big around as he was tall. He had no sense of balance and couldn't even sit up. He was like a Weeble, but he did fall down. The Boy had no neck at all. His head just rested on his shoulders. What a sight. But here is the interesting thing. He stayed at the same weight for two years, and just grew tall. He's probably the only baby that wore out his clothes. But as The Boy grew into his toddlerhood, I noticed a total lack of pattern in his eating. I couldn't force The Boy to eat if my life depended on it. I remember one day being at the pool with my friend Anne, and the following conversation took place: We're sitting on the side of the baby pool watching our two three-year old sons playing in the water:

"So what did The Boy have for dinner last night?" says Anne.

"Nothing, followed by a Popsicle for dessert."

What I did find was my son was very good at listening to his body for what nutrition he needed. As a toddler, he almost never sat down to a real meal. He would eat food on the go. He would have an orange here, a glass of milk there, half a ham sandwich. I began to realize that he was amazingly good at bringing perfect nutrition into his body when I allowed him to listen to himself. I did sway him by giving him choices. If I had taken the time to write down all the food he ate over the course of a week, it would probably look like some sort of funky version of the food pyramid. To this day my son, who is twenty-two years old, really has a good sense of what his body needs. He has a gorgeous body, but he absolutely never stresses about food. For him, he knows it's all good.

My son simply has never allowed any of the lies and white noise come into his psyche about food. He most definitely does not suffer from SWAD. To him food is good, and that's all you need to know. He enjoys moving his body and working out at the gym, and aspires to be a personal trainer and fitness expert. But what really sets him apart at this point, is his total commitment to common sense. He has not begun micromanaging every morsel he puts in his mouth. He eats, he enjoys, and he moves his body, simple common sense.

Here's another thing. Ever since I was a kid, I was told that breakfast was the most important meal of the day. My mother pounded into us that you had to eat a good healthy breakfast before heading off to school or your brain won't function properly and you'd be a failure as a human being. What a load to bear when I CAN'T EAT IN THE MORNING! I don't remember a time when eating first thing in the morning was something I wanted to do. It literally makes me feel sick to my stomach to eat in the morning. My body doesn't want food in the morning. My mother made us breakfast every school day morning, and she didn't scrimp either. Eggs and bacon, waffles, pancakes, oatmeal, and occasionally we would get what I consider to be the crème de la crème of breakfast...fruit cocktail. She and I battled over my not wanting to eat breakfast for years. I think she finally gave up when I lied and told her I could get a roll or something at the cafeteria in middle school.

I am a morning person. I wake up like a shot most mornings, and I am well into my day before I even get my slippers on. I think best in the morning, and have historically saved a vast majority of my thinking tasks for the morning time. If breakfast was the most important meal of the day, and this was true of every person in the whole world, I would think my body would be accommodating this. Yet it doesn't. I don't think we can correlate the opposite way either. I don't think I think worse when there is food in my stomach. I think the presence or absence of food has nothing to do with how my brain operates on a daily basis. I believe my brain functionality is on a rhythmic schedule that has nothing to do with food. However, with that said, if you deprive your body of food for a long term, it will affect your brain, as well as all of your other organs.

I will acquiesce that my body functions better when I'm fed. A few days ago, I had skipped breakfast, as always, and in the early afternoon I grabbed a small snack rather than having a real lunch. When I came back upstairs to work, I wanted to do a bouncy ball dance party. I started the party, but found that I was really very tired and didn't want to do it too much. So I stopped. I hadn't slept well the night before and figured this was the reason. I went on with my day writing, and called it quits later in the afternoon. After dinner I wanted to have another bouncy ball dance party, so I went upstairs and got out my headset and ball, and sure enough I had a really great dance party. I was full of energy, and the difference was that I ate a good dinner and was feeling excellent. My body was telling me earlier in the afternoon that I hadn't eaten enough to sustain a party. When we turn off the white noise of the obsessing over food and exercise, and allow ourselves to hear our bodies, the wisdom of our nature comes shining through. It is time to recapture the wisdom.

May 12, 2011

Yesterday was an epiphany day for me. I began reading Eckhart Tolle's A New Earth and have both confirmed my theory of collective madness and have expanded upon it. For those of you who may not be familiar with Eckhart Tolle, he is an advanced thought and spiritual leader. He has been on Oprah Winfrey's show many times. Anyway, I think for the first time in my life I am finally finding some peace on the topic of weight.

I believe one of the most important things to have come out of my studying Tolle is the return to the egoless state. Eckhart Tolle talks of the collective madness that humanity has fallen into in the last two hundred years or so. He does acknowledge, and I agree with him that madness has always been around, but it was sporadic. There would be a war here and a war there, and maybe the Crusades, etc., but widespread and constant madness was not the norm until beginning maybe two hundred years ago.

However the madness I am most interested in is the war we have waged on our own bodies. For the purposes of this book I am going to concentrate on weight as the issue, but overall health is another issue for another book.

It seems at some point in history the human ego took possession of how our bodies look and how we as humans perceive how our bodies look. Prior this time period, body image is something that simply didn't exist. You had a body and that was the end of it. I have to believe that mirrors either hadn't been invented yet, or they were the exclusive domain of the rich or royals. During these times it is fair to say that most people never really saw a reflection of themselves across their entire lifetime. Without being able to see their own image, they had no idea what their face or body looked like. Oh sure they could see their own hair if it grew long enough, and they could look down and see their bodies, but the preoccupation into what they looked like simply did not exist. The ego had not yet taken possession of the care and upkeep of the human body. The human body was on auto pilot. Nature gave us a perfect human body and we lived with it until it was no longer perfect and it was time to shed it. Early planned obsolescence.

But then something happened, something that drew humans, and probably the rich or royal with means to spend, to the more aesthetic. It was probably during a particularly good economic time when working for material goods wasn't necessary for the upper class, and to fill time, they turned their attention to more hedonistic things like sex and beauty. Sex, beauty, art, food, literature...all good things to be sure, until the ego takes hold of them. Suddenly "improvement" of one's features became important. Women bought corsets and brassieres to shape and hold naturally occurring body parts in ways that are unnatural to the human body, just to conjure up an illusion or an image of a perfect body. Image is never one hundred percent accurate and illusion can tell many lies.

May 17, 2011

It seems to me that from what I can understand about Ego, we can't completely get away from it as human beings. It is extremely entrenched into us after thousands of years of existence. Recognizing it, and acknowledging it, and even minimizing it, is a gift in and of itself. So I am well versed in the idea that the ego is what is running this weight show we have going on here.

Since I started the bouncy ball dance parties, one of the things I've begun noticing is that my appetite has returned. I'm not going to go into this whole thing with metabolism and all, that's been done to death. I do believe that because for the first time in a very long time, because I'm enjoying how I'm moving my body, my body is enjoying being with me too. My appetite is so much better, and I want to eat more. My body is metabolizing the food perfectly and I feel myself getting thinner and thinner all the time. The more I'm enjoying myself, body-wise, the more my body is giving me to enjoy. When I was at my peak weight, I wasn't enjoying myself at all, and I had absolutely no appetite. The food I did eat wasn't enjoyable either.

If the goal is happiness, then why are so many people obese and unhappy? It's because we collectively allowed our ego to guide the decisions about our bodies. We decided that after tens of thousands of years where nature took care of our weight, we were going to control it once and for all. Ego has done a terrible job. If we can drop our ego and allow nature to return us to our natural weight by moving our bodies in a way that feels good, we will get there and get there quickly. When I was finally able to let go, and understand that all of the control I've been exercising over my body has resulted in worse and worse results, the more relaxed I've become. I understand right now that I'm beautiful just because I exist. I have covered up the mirrors in the house, and only use them sparingly. For the sake of sanity and the ability to continue forward encouraged, I do not look at my reflection in the mirror. I feel better and look better without looking in the mirror.

SHOW BUSINESS

Last night I went with some friends to see a play which was playing at a local theatre. One of the stars of the production was a former cast member from a long running soap opera that is now off the air. In her role on the soap opera she was quite the siren. Her character was long suffering, yet seemed to either sleep with or marry every available and unavailable man on the show. I hadn't watched the show in maybe twenty years, but was loosely aware that she was on it until the end.

Before the curtain I looked over the Play Bill and saw her familiar picture and biography. I had seen her on other shows before, so I was looking forward to her live performance. When she came out, I was somewhat stunned at how much weight she had gained over the last time I had seen her on television. I wasn't so much stunned by her weight as I was about how different her appearance was compared to the picture in the Play Bill. I would have adjusted to her change in appearance except for one thing. She couldn't hide her discomfort. As an actress she executed her role beautifully, and she was funny and her timing was impeccable. Yet, seemingly absent mindedly, she fussed with her wardrobe in a very familiar way (covering the gut bulge) almost constantly throughout the performance.

In a song and dance number which was her time to shine, her discomfort was so clear, as she was picked up and put down on props by a group of handsome male cast members. I was in pain for her. Because of her weight she simply could not completely get into character. I've never seen this before. This is not a testament to the fact that she is a bad actress. Not at all, she is a very good actress with multiple Emmy Awards, and a resume that any working actor would want. No, this is a testament to what The Cult has done.

May 31, 2011

Sucked back in big time.

The epiphanies keep coming. It's been awhile since I've written a word on this topic, but I have been living it and thinking it. It continues to astound me how far from nature we have really come. It is still surprising me. One of the things that has been evolving out of my new thinking, or reverting back to old thinking, is the last time we were all naturally at our perfect weight was when we walked everywhere. There were markets to go to, not Super Grocery Centers. Back in the day my mom would stock up on certain items weekly at the supermarket, such as toiletry items, paper goods, laundry detergent, and whatnot. Sure she would pick up some frozen items, breakfast cereal, and food for our school lunches, but fresh food was bought daily. Meats, vegetables and dairy products were all bought on a daily, or near daily basis.

I remember when I was a little kid; seasonal fruit was such a treat. In the summer, on our way home from the pool, there was a fruit stand. The owner of the fruit stand, Bert, carried the best seasonal fruit. I could smell the watermelons and peaches when we pulled up in the car. My mother would stop at the stand and we would pick out peaches and nectarines, and the most amazing New Jersey sweet white corn. We could hardly wait to get home to have a peach for a snack. They were so ripe and delicious and juicy, my mother made us eat the peaches outside. What a great snack. I believe with the mass introduction of the USDA Food Pyramid, enjoyment of our fruits and vegetables became a chore.

I grew up eating fruits and vegetables. Fresh when they were seasonal and canned when they were not seasonally available. But as soon as science was introduced into my diet, and nature was taken away, eating according to science became a bore. I don't want to be told I have to eat fruits and vegetables. That is a recipe for my wanting chips and cookies. Before food became mandatory I enjoyed fruits and vegetables, and often took veggies out of the refrigerator and ate them raw for a snack. Not because they were "good" foods, but because I liked them. I can only speak for myself, but as soon as the consumption became mandatory I pushed back with foods that were considered to be off limits. Honestly what happens when you try to control a teenager? They rebel.

With The Cult trying to control every aspect of our dietary lives, there is no doubt we were going to rebel, but look at the insanity of the rebellion. We rebel against the food pyramid and eat at McDonalds. We rebel against the weight/height charts. At one point in history we were free range humans. We ate according to our own nature. But then The Cult began telling us what to do and what to eat, and we rebelled against the control. Then we gain weight and stop moving around, and the bad feelings about being fat send us to the other side of The Cult, who tells us it is mandatory to exercise and curb your appetite, and we try to do that too. When that level of control fails, we rebel again to eating whatever we want while sticking out our tongue, and then get fat again, and so on and so on.

I'm now walking for utility as much as the weather will allow. I walk to the store daily to get food for dinner. Today I walked to a fruit and vegetable market I had never been to before and bought beautiful seasonal fruit for snacking. I couldn't believe the difference between this fruit and what I find at the grocery store. I walked to my favorite deli and got a sandwich for lunch.

Looking back at those times when I was naturally thin, even the last time when I had a mixed result because I was doing an abdominal workout that I didn't like, there was one common thread involved. I walked for about two hours a day. When I was a teen, the two hours comprised the time it took to walk to school and home. I didn't do it all at once, but I did walk a minimum of two hours a day. I didn't power walk, I transportation walked. When my daughter was a baby and I had no car, my daily errands took me about two hours a day. In this case I actually did it all at the same time because The Girl was a baby and I wanted the errands done before her nap. Again, I didn't power walk, but transportation walked, as I was pushing a stroller. The last time I walked an hour in the morning with one dog, and an hour in the afternoon with the other. I may have been pressing the walk a little harder because the dogs like to go faster, and I was deliberately walking to lose weight....weight that I promptly gained back when I "finished."

There should be no "finished" with this. Walking is nature's way to keep us naturally thin. Have we morphed into a time obsessed society? Yes. I know many of you will look at my words and shake your head and call me a fraud because I'm suggesting, at least for myself, that I have to move my body a minimum of two hours a day. But here is the beauty of this truth, I only have to move my body for a couple hours a day to resume my perfect state of natural thinness. Once I'm there, listening for what my body needs in terms of movement, and responding accordingly is all I need to stay thin. Remember, when I was a teen, I was naturally thin, and stayed that way even after I began driving a car. I was still moving my body, but I didn't need to do it two hours a day. I am simply in a temporary place where I need to assist my body in finding its perfect state of natural slenderness and health. Once I return there maintaining will be easy and intuitive. Just like when I was a child. No struggle. No measure, nothing. Just simply existing inside my perfect body and enjoying my life.

So where does this leave the bouncy ball dance parties? Exactly where they are today. Bouncy ball dance parties are a great way to move the body and a fun way to melt your middle. Bouncy ball dance parties are celebratory, and I suggest you do one every day. It makes your body feel good and it makes your spirit feel good, and it's something you can do with friends. It is dancing, and dancing is natural and normal for human beings. It does not replace walking, but is a fun addition to walking.

June 9, 2011

Hey it's me again. Just keep reading. Do not follow what I say. Understand that this is me wrestling my way out of The Cult.

It is about a year and a week since I began writing this book, and when I look back over the struggle this last year has been, in terms of coming to some sort of understanding about weight and the issue it has become not only for me, but worldwide, has been eye opening. Because I have had to go down this road alone without council, it has been a very long and lonely road. I find when I try to talk some sense into people about what it is I'm discovering, there seems to be a sparkle in their eyes, momentarily. I seem to be hitting people with the remembrance of what is used to be, and they agree that it wasn't like this at all, but then they go right back into the party line. It's almost like talking to a member of a weird religious cult, and for a slight second there is that moment of clarity, that moment where you see the actual person inside emerge, and then retreat behind the brainwashing again. Too afraid to take personal responsibility for the state they find themselves in. Happy in the notion that they are not to be blamed and that surely at some point, The Fat Cult will bring the perfect diet to them, at long last.

But I do know I'm onto something here. I do know that whatever the answer to this problem is, it's incredibly simple. I understand that the two times in my life that I was totally and naturally thin was when I walked with purpose and utility. I keep trying to make that work for me, but the problem became that I put rules and numbers around it. Only a few entries ago I was spouting about how I have to walk for at least two hours a day. There we go, another rule I put on myself. I am so used to prescription movement that I actually take out the prescription pad and write them for myself now.

A year and six days after beginning writing this book I am still struggling to get out of The Cult. This is how destructive and all-encompassing it is. A year and six days ago I had an intellectual concept of what is going wrong with the world when it comes to the topic of weight and health, and the emotional component has been so strong that I am still struggling to get out, in spite of my intellectual understanding. I believe I am almost there. I will keep journaling this to let you know. I have come to realize that I do not need to have two hours of "movement" a day. I walk for utility and purpose, and that's it. When I can I do, when I can't I don't. No counting. No guilt. My perfect natural thinness is coming to me because I am finally respecting the honest and true nature of how my body is designed, and my body is responding in kind. Simple as that, right? Then why has it been so hard for me to grasp these concepts? Because I am so absolutely, totally brainwashed by The Cult. This fucking sucks.

July 4, 2011

This is my favorite chapter so far. I finally do make some sense here.

So I'm out walking today with my dog Lily. She is an amazing walking partner. There are things that I thought about that began to make an awful lot of sense. One of them is the notion that we are so egotistical both collectively and individually that we think that we can control our weight. I've said it before and I'll say it again, that which you fight most against, is what you attract. The war on drugs which started as a war on illegal street drugs has morphed into a problem with prescription drugs, and even over-the-counter drugs. There are doctors out there that just write prescriptions to people for them to sell on the street. College students are taking Adderall, an ADD medication to "help" them study. The problem with prescription drug abuse is worse than the problem with illegal street drugs now. Hell, there are people out there smoking bath salts! Talk about Calgon take me away! We are fighting and we cannot possibly win. Did no one learn anything from Prohibition?

The same goes with our Fight against Obesity. We are attracting nothing but more obesity.

As I've already covered, our bodies are designed as flawlessly as something that is destined for the junk heap can be. We are born with all of the mechanisms for good health naturally. We are born with the natural ability to determine what foods are good for us without the benefit of anyone telling us what to eat. Before the media, individuals and families made decisions about nutrition without as much as a thought. They ate meat that was hunted, and locally and seasonally available fruits and vegetables. There was no food pyramid, and no height weight charts. Nowhere in history is there reference to a society that was overweight, nowhere. Man, in his evolution, invented ways to manipulate these food products into other food products that are also delicious and nutritious. Foods such as cheese, and bread, even wine and beer, which are made from multiple ingredients. This makes the consumption of food not only utilitarian and necessary, but wonderful and sensuous. Our bodies have the mechanism to tell us when to eat, and when to stop eating because we've had enough. Our bodies are built for movement, both in a utilitarian way and also in joyful ways.

But what have we done in our crazy ego driven state? We have denied all of the mechanisms naturally built into our bodies that regulate weight, in favor of what we have determined is best. This goes completely against the sheer nature of our bodies. Who are we to do this? We were already born with perfection. Let me see if I can demonstrate how irrational human kind has become on this topic.

Let's stop talking about weight and talk about body temperature instead. This is a good jumping off point. We all know that the average person's internal body temperature is 98.6 degrees Fahrenheit. When I was a kid, and I got a temperature above 98.6 mom automatically gave me a baby aspirin to lower it. Luckily science has discovered that automatically medicating a slightly elevated temperature is a bad idea. The reason the human body runs a temperature is to fight off disease. A person with a 101-102 degree temperature is cooking out a foreign and unwanted virus or bacteria. Medicating and bringing down the body temperature could result in the virus or bacteria being able to take foothold, and cause damage to the body. Luckily science figured this out, and we only begin medicating a temperature when it gets to the danger point, around 103 or higher. At that temperature the body could be in serious trouble if it is left alone for long.

Mind you the reason this discovery was made fairly easily was because having an elevated body temperature has nothing to do with the ego. One doesn't judge another or themselves based on their body temperature. In fact 98.6 is the average body temperature, but not necessarily for everyone. Some people are naturally above or below that temperature, and this says absolutely nothing about them as a person. It is just normal for them. Normal. Now, I'm going to put the same spin on body temperature that humankind in its ultimate wisdom put on weight. Let's just say that the actress Julia Roberts remarks in an interview that her normal body temperature is one hundred degrees. That's it. She doesn't say anything more, other than her normal body temperature is one hundred degrees. Remember Twiggy back in the

1960's....she didn't say anything at all. She was just really thin, which was natural and normal for her body.

Taking the Julia Roberts scenario further, through the use of the Internet, The National Enquirer, TMZ and People Magazine, everyone on the planet has heard that Julia Roberts has a body temperature of one hundred degrees. People begin to correlate that a one hundred degree body temperature equals a beautiful, thin, successful person with an amazing life and career. What happens next? Products to elevate body temperature begin to hit the market. Spas that cater to elevating your temperature dot the landscape. Young girls taunt each other with "You're cold," which sends them into a heating disorder. Millions of people become addicted to heat pills, and maintain their body temperatures at one hundred degrees, and it becomes a fashion statement to wear a thermometer around your neck at all times. New areas of medicine are identified such as Heatiatrics and Heatiology, which studies the phenomena of organ melting. People begin going deaf by the hundreds of thousands because ear wax is melting and oozing out, allowing dangerous bacteria into the ear canal. People are dying of organ meltdowns and brain fry, and instead of looking at the source of the problem, we keep looking for solutions to the symptoms until small children are suffering from organ meltdown and brain fry, and life expectancy begins to drop throughout society. In our collective damaged ego, we have allowed our "knowledge" to override our nature. Nature always wins.

July 7, 2011

...and I get sucked back in

Today was a big day for me in terms of epiphany. My day began at 3:00 this morning when I woke up and had difficulty getting back to sleep. I had a dental appointment scheduled for first thing this morning which I was dreading, causing me some anxiety. For the next three hours I was up and down, going to the bathroom and getting back in bed only to toss and turn. To say it was a very frustrating three hours is an understatement. I finally got out of bed and started my day cranky and fussy, and seriously not looking forward to my dental appointment.

I came downstairs and pondered why it was that I couldn't sleep. And why was it that the night before I slept like a baby? I mean I did wake up once during the night, at five o'clock in the morning to go to the bathroom, but then fell right back to sleep when I returned to bed. What was the issue?

The difference between my sleep last night, and my sleep the night before, was the level of activity I engaged in. The day before yesterday I walked with my dogs in the morning, and then walked to and from the bank. I had a bouncy ball dance party in the afternoon, and then walked with my dogs again after dinner. My body had actually had enough activity to promote a good night sleep. Yesterday I walked to work, but that was it in terms of activity. My body was telling me, by waking me up at 3:00 in the morning that I had not moved my body enough. That's it, my whole epiphany. I do believe my body will return it its natural state of perfect thinness when I honor its wishes and get enough activity to foster a good night rest. Then in the morning I will wake refreshed and ready to engage in more physical and intellectual activity. The key is balance. Eat in moderation, move your body accordingly, and sleep peacefully. The cycle is perfection. It's a matter of honoring it.

July 8, 2011

I am amazed at the pervasiveness of The Cult. Just when I had the thoughts I thought in the last post, my mind began racing again. More movement is better than less, and I began going right back into the obsessive thinking patterns that have only served to keep me fat. I have been writing this book, and trying to live it for thirteen months now, and I'm not much closer to my perfect weight now than I was thirteen months ago. I have been walking and doing my dance parties to no avail. Last night I thought about what my day today was going to be like and thought it would be a good idea to get up at 5:30 in the morning so I could walk with the dogs before I went to work. Now mind you, I have just theorized that moving the body to the point of being tired at the end of the day was my goal. So is it reasonable to deliberately interrupt sleep in order to get up so I can be tired? That makes no sense at all. Not to mention, I don't like getting up that early. My body resists it every time. It was that old sense of obligation, of guilt, of "If I don't do it at 5:30 in the morning when am I going to do it?" It is absolutely astonishing to me how deep the talons of The Cult go, when I have been working on this issue for thirteen months and I still default back to the flawed thinking that has kept me on this treadmill (pardon the pun) for thirteen months....actually for thirty years!

This morning I got out of bed and saw the neat pile of workout clothes and my sneakers sitting on my dresser waiting for my 5:30 wake up call, which didn't happen. Why do I have to keep making the same mistakes over and over again? Why is my thinking so dangerously flawed? Because I've been systematically trained, just like you, to live in and accept the lies.

...do not take copious notes.

The Keys to Your New Life

Today, July 8, 2011 I was finally able to see what has eluded me for thirty years. This is it. I hope you're ready. Take out a paper and pen and be prepared to take copious notes. The key to returning to your state of natural thinness is this: Eat whatever you like in moderation and balance your diet with delicious and varied foods. 2) Move your body in ways that you enjoy to the point of inducing a perfect state of sleep at the end of the day.

Up until today I understood about the eating, I had already nailed it. I understood moving my body in ways that I like. Here is where I got all tripped up. I kept thinking in terms of weight loss. If you think about weight, you get weight. It doesn't matter if you're thinking about loss or gain, you will get weight. Here is where I made my simple turn of thought that worked out perfectly. Up until now I thought of moving my body as "exercise" which I have stated before is a prescription term. When I was a kid we didn't exercise we played. The difference was we really enjoyed what we did. Thinking about when I was going to fit in exercise caused stress in me because exercise is not something I want to do, and fitting in something I don't want to do in the course of my day is extremely stressful. It's sort of like putting off going to the dentist until the pain gets overwhelming. You will say you don't have time until the pain is so bad, time is irrelevant. So for me, everything came before "exercising" because I hated it that much. This morning I had a complete change of thinking that is going to change everything about how I approach moving my body and achieving the perfect sense of peace and tiredness at the end of the day.

This is what it is: I ask myself during the course of my day, "What do I feel like doing that is fun and will make me tired at the end of the day?" Notice I didn't say a word about weight? Suddenly I have time. I have time to do fun things. I love walking, so I walked back and forth to work. This afternoon I'm going to have a bouncy ball dance party, and after dinner I will treat my dogs to a nice half hour walk each before showering and ending my day. I also ordered a dorky looking tricycle for myself so I can tool around and go to the food store, or just to take for a nice ride. I have weather proofed this too. I have a treadmill, so I can listen to books on my mp3 player while taking a walk. I do my bouncy ball dance parties, and I really love doing those. I have dance parties on game console that I enjoy as well.

When I woke up this morning I didn't realize that I would be finishing the book today. That today was the day I was going to arrive at this most simple epiphany. It is my hope that through my words that many of you can skip the steps of struggling to get out of The Cult, although I think that those of you who can remember life before the pandemic spread of fat will have an easier time. For those of you who cannot see a world where people were naturally thin, please listen to me now, it was.

July 23, 2011

A corner is being turned...

Today is a magical day. Many things that I need to know became absolutely apparent today. I've received one good idea after the next. The Universe has really worked against me in terms of allowing me to move my body in the ways that I like. The weather has been awful. It's been a very hot few weeks, and I haven't been able to walk or even ride my bike. The other day I went upstairs to do a bouncy ball dance party, and my headphones snapped in half. It seems to me that the Universe was trying to tell me something. What it is trying to get me to understand more than anything else I've discovered in the last fourteen months is the organ between our ears is more responsible for our weight than anything we eat, or any way we move our bodies. I am still giving negative attention to my abdomen, and this is why I continue to be heavy. It is time that I replace my negative thoughts with positive thin thoughts.

I will stop using the word weight, because using the word weight will only attract weight. I am using the word thin, and I expect to be attracting thin from this moment on. I will practice the art of non-judgment and when I see someone with less thinness than me, I will replace the image with a thin one. I will act kindly to myself and know that my thinness is on its way, it's just a matter of my having the right mind set. While moving our bodies is good for the structure, and is helpful in keeping our form and brain balanced, it is the power of our thoughts that will make us thin and keep us thin. We must become a society where weight is no longer an issue. We must return to our own nature, where nature determined our body style and perfect weight, not us flawed human beings. So far we've fouled it up pretty bad. I know I have.

As I allow the notion of thin thoughts to sink into my psyche, I think back on the two times in my life I was perfectly naturally thin. When I was a teenager, and when I had no car and had to walk everywhere. Here is what I'm gleaning from these two times. When I was a teen, I was perfectly naturally thin, and simply didn't think about it. It was normal for me. It just wasn't something I thought about at all. I didn't think about the food I ate or what I didn't eat, or amounts or anything. It was a non-issue. Interestingly, when I walked with the stroller because I didn't have a car, I KNEW I was going to get rail thin, and I got rail thin. But when I got a car again, I KNEW I was going to gain weight and I did. Now I am putting it in my mind that now that I have a perfect understanding of how this works, I'm simply going to allow myself to return to my perfect thin state, and then I will assume that I am going to stay there forever. No other effort required. I will move my body according to what I feel like doing and do it joyfully. I will enjoy my walks with my dogs because it's something I love doing. I will simply allow my body to resume its perfection beginning now and never think about it again. Done.

The fact of the matter is you cannot attract good when you feel bad. If you feel bad about your body then you absolutely cannot attract a beautiful body. The reason I was able to be perfectly thin all of the times I did it, was because there was always one of two things occurring. First, there was a complete absence of any thoughts about weight. Weight was neither good nor bad, it just was. Or, secondly, there was the belief that I was going to be at a certain weight. When I had to walk with my baby to run errands, I believed that I was going to be thin, so my thoughts were of thinness, not weight, and voila, I got thin. Then my belief shifted to believing that because I was no longer walking everywhere, that I was going to gain weight, and voila, I gained weight. It is up to me to eliminate all fat thoughts from my mind and get to the point where I never even think about weight, and I will naturally fall right back into the default factory settings that my body should be, with no effort at all on my part.

Knowing this is an amazing gift. I am blessed to have figured this out. Now it's a matter of finally and completely rejecting The Cult from my life because the level of mind control they have had over me is astonishing. It may take a great deal of my energy moving forward but I'm going to do it. I may also ask for an assist from my ego to push it through. I am going to posit that once my body begins to show signs of normalizing; looking in the mirror to see the results will be a good thing. Seeing beautiful results will encourage me to think even more thin thoughts, and allow me to get excited about my thinning body which will lead to more thin thoughts. Right now I'm faking it until I make it, but once I do make it, I am going to think thin thoughts all of the time, which will zoom it to me faster and faster, until at last, one day, the fat thoughts will simply stop being an issue at all.

July 26, 2011

Today I am three weeks shy of the official launch of my book *Unemployed: How Desperation Led Me to the Worst Job ever.* I'm pretty busy dealing with details and whatnot on steps that need to be done before the official launch. Yesterday I had a meeting with The Social Guru, who advises me on all things social networking including my website. She suggested that I stick some sort of tagline into a blank space on the top of the homepage. This morning that tagline came to me. I'm quoting me on this because I made it up. "The absence of thought defaults perfection."

The absence of thought defaults perfection. What does that mean exactly? It means that I have hit on the holy grail of the obesity problem. Before The Cult existed there was no thought of our bodies, of their size or weight. It wasn't thought about and it wasn't discussed. It just was what it was. Our bodies tended to default to their perfect weight because we simply did not think about it. Just like in my example about controlling our internal body temperature. We don't think about it and it defaults to its own perfection. Thinking thin thoughts is not going to work either because you will always be chasing thin. Thinking no thoughts about weight is the only way to normalize it perfectly, and for the last time. Moving your body does not normalize your weight, it is just another cog in the wheel of keeping you healthy. My mother never moved her body at all when I was a kid. She didn't think about her weight either. She was a perfect 100 pounds at all times. Not moving her body did contribute to health problems such as arthritis, but now that she's older she is moving her body every day and feels better than ever. She doesn't think about her weight at all and she remains perfectly trim. Moving her body has only helped to improve her health.

Getting out of the grips of The Cult has been a very long road for me, but mostly because I've been figuring this out by myself. I do believe that with this knowledge we can crawl out from under The Cult's control and take our bodies back perfectly and naturally. Never diet and exercise again. Eat and allow the food to perfectly metabolize into our bodies. Remember, back when there were no fat people we ate whatever we wanted. As a society we were relatively disease free. The word "cancer" was whispered. No one knew what diabetes was, it was that rare. Allow food to metabolize into your body perfectly. Don't even think about it.

Now, you're going to ask me how we change how we're thinking about this. Well it's going to be a process, but I'll walk us through it. As you can see through the course of this book I have been on a process myself. It has taken me more than thirteen months to work this through, to figure it out. Finally I have figured it out. Here is what we know:

- Trying to control our weight has been a massive failure. Just like trying to control our body temperature, this is an exercise in futility. Our bodies are born with the default mechanism to be perfectly naturally slender.
- Food does not make us fat; thinking about weight makes us fat
- Diets are a recipe for failure. You are set up to think about lack of food, which sets you up for feeling a lack of food, which makes food an enemy. Food is just food. It doesn't possess a goodness or badness.
- Stop counting. Counting and tabulating causes stress. Stress is not good. If you aren't feeling good you cannot possibly attract goodness to you. This is why diets fail. Diets, no matter what kind, even the "all chocolate" diet doesn't feel good.
- Eat what you like in moderation. Nothing is off limits. Food is only food. There are no good foods or bad foods. There are only good thoughts and bad thoughts.
- Move your body every day. It isn't necessary for your perfect thinness because I know lots of people who are thin and couch potatoes. Moving your body is essential to your good health and well-being, and honestly it makes you feel good when it's an activity you enjoy.

Remember that this is a process and it takes time to deprogram from the lies we've been told. I have been working this issue actively, every single day since June 3, 2010. It has taken every ounce of my will to push through the lies. These lies have been so greatly ingrained into my psyche, just when I think I have a concept nailed, BLAM! I tithe to the beast, or fall for the pretty words "flat abs fast." Recognize that we have been brainwashed into thinking that we were the ones that had to control this and be a body type and style that our bodies are not meant to be. Everyone is born with a default body. I know my default body is around one hundred and eighteen pounds. I will never get on a scale again, but that is what I recall my body defaulting to. However, if my body, in its return to factory settings, turns out to be more Reubenesque, then so be it. I am perfect. You are perfect. Allow it.

Relinquish control. That which we seek to control ends up controlling us. If you are trying to be skinny, you will always have to be trying to be skinny. If you are trying to lose weight, you are always going to be trying to lose weight. If you are simply perfect, then the perfect body you were born with will appear in record time.

How do I get these thoughts out of my head, you ask? This is an exercise that will shock and surprise you. You will need to listen to your emotions. When you give negative feedback to yourself in the form of a thought, it feels bad. Replace that thought immediately with "I'm perfect." Any thought that makes you cringe, replace it with "I'm perfect. What will shock you is how often every day you will find yourself saying "I'm perfect." However, in that simplicity, you will be attracting your perfect default factory settings body. The trick is to be happy with it when it comes. Don't look at someone else and decide you want a body like them. You can't have it. You've already proven it with a lifetime of diet and exercise. It is as silly as me going on a stretching plan to grow longer legs so I can have legs like Christie Brinkley. I simply cannot accomplish it by trying to control my height.

Understand that until the last couple hundred years, our human form has self-regulated without any assistance from us. There was no food pyramid. People ate what was indigenous to their land. We have moved so far away from our own nature, that many can't even see it. Like I said earlier, the people that will grapple the hardest with these concepts are those that never saw a world that wasn't obese. I do remember a world where the word "diversity" could mean different shapes and sizes, and everyone was okay with that. There was a time when absolutely no one stressed about weight, and we are now on the cusp of returning back to that time. What a blessing.

July 28, 2011

Hello Cult! Good to see you!

My thoughts continue to evolve. One of the things that have been haunting me is how often my thoughts go negative as it comes to my body. Not even my entire body, basically my abdominal area. I pay more negative attention there than I do anywhere else. Actually that is the only area that I find fault with. I am forever tugging on my pants, trying to find a comfortable place on my waistline for my pants to rest. The thing I've been struggling with is these negative messages and how they're holding me back, and how I must stop thinking these fat thoughts. I had a revelation this morning. I thought back on those two times in my life that I was perfectly thin and put together those things that correlated together, and this is what I came up with. When I was a teenager, I struck a perfect balance in weight because I 1) never thought about weight at all; 2) ate whatever I wanted whenever I wanted to; 3) moved my body in ways that were functional and fun; 4) enjoyed looking at myself in the mirror. When I was a young mother this is what happened: 1) thought about being thin; 2) ate whatever I wanted whenever I wanted to; 3) moved my body in a way that was functional; 4) enjoyed looking at myself in the mirror.

This is where I am today: 1) All I think about is fat; 2) eat whatever I want whenever I want to; 3) don't move my body much; 4) horrified by what I see in the mirror. I'm still 184 pounds, I think. So now what? What do I do with this? Here is what I am proposing, and I'll let you know how it works for me. One of the things that have me so stuck is how to stop giving myself bad messages. I am going to go ahead and say something that I normally wouldn't say. I am going to engage my ego for good purposes. Generally speaking ego holds us down and keeps us in negativity. I am going to re-engage in daily movement. I am going to move my body by riding my ridiculous tricycle, walking with my dogs, or doing the bouncy ball dance parties. I have determined how much time I need to do this for my body to be tired at the end of the day. I am not going to fight my fat thoughts at all. Let 'em rip I say. Because once I begin behaving the way I did when I was a young mother and a teenager, my body will naturally begin to take its perfect shape, and the bad thoughts will go away. Once my shape begins to return, I will begin looking in the mirror again, and admire my beautiful new body, which will only lead me to thinking more thin thoughts, which will lead me to more mirror gazing and more thin thoughts.

The fact of the matter is that if we are overweight, it is our body's way of telling us that something is wrong and to fix it. Being fat isn't wrong; it is simply a symptom that something is out of whack. Just like running a temperature means that you are fighting off disease. Gaining weight is simply a symptom, not a disease. You will return to your perfect natural weight easily and effortlessly when you identify how to enjoy moving your body, and doing it enough to make you tired like a little kid. You can eat what you like, when you like it, in moderate portions. When I say moderate portions, please understand that feeling full is not an indicator that you've eaten enough. Just like being thirsty isn't an indicator that your body needs fluids. Eat a modest portion at every meal and you can always eat whatever you want. This includes snacks too.

So remember, being overweight is just a symptom that your life is out of balance. Correct the balance and your perfect body will return easily. You will never diet and exercise again a day in your life once that balance is struck, and you will never have to spend another dime for the privilege.

September 3, 2011

...and I get out of The Cult yet again, but on a limited level

Today was yet another epiphany. It's been a day full of them. But I am going to stay on track with the whole weight issue. I know for a fact now that what I'm being asked to do is to use the power of my mind to return to my natural weight. No more bouncy ball dance parties. That would be just yet another form of exercise that dupes people into thinking that this will solve their weight issues, when in fact; one hundred percent of it is between the ears. Beginning today I am going to journal or visualize for fifteen minutes a day about what I want my body to look like, and every Monday I am going to take a picture of me to compare with the week before. I believe because of my level of excitement about this, and my realization that this is going to happen quickly, it will happen quickly. I know that this is happening and I have turned a very key corner. I am on the path of most allowance. I am so happy about this that all thoughts of fat and negativity have left my brain and I am just thinking about how thin I'm about to be. No more bouncy ball. It is time for me to use the power of my brain and do this deliberately. I know the time is finally right because up until this moment I have resisted vigorously the idea of documenting my progress. But now I am going to take pictures of my body and weigh myself every Saturday beginning today. No matter what the scale says it's fine because it is just going to go down, down, down until I rest at the perfect weight for my body. This is very exciting! I'm leaving now for my husband's chiropractic office to weigh myself and get a steno pad.

I'm back. In the process of writing this book for the last fifteen months, I haven't dieted, but I have exercised quite a bit. Thousands of hours of walking with my dogs and bouncy ball dance parties, and guess what? I gained nine pounds. I weigh more now than I ever have. I am a whopping one hundred and ninety three pounds. Conventional wisdom, in terms of what is popularly believed, says that I should have lost a lot of weight. I eat very little and I exercised a lot, but yet I gained weight. I was writing about weight, and what I got was more weight. It doesn't matter that I was talking about returning to a good weight, I was thinking about weight, so I got nine more pounds because nature figured, if that's what I'm thinking about, then clearly it is something I love and want, so it gave me more of what I was thinking about. This is over now. I know what needs to be done.

To get to my perfect weight of one hundred and eighteen pounds, I will need to shed seventy five pounds, the most I've ever had to take off in my life. I have literally gone from my perfect weight of one hundred and eighteen pounds to one hundred and ninety three pounds. I have gained a 5th grader.

Moving forward I am going to document daily what I eat, so you all can see that I'm not dieting. I have stopped any sort of deliberate exercise, although walking with my dogs is something I will do with them, weather permitting. I will weigh myself weekly, and let me tell you this is something I have feared all these years. However, I am so confident that my body will return to its natural thinness by using the power of my thoughts, and the use of journaling and visualization, that the results will be astonishing. I'll check back in when I'm at 118 pounds.

October 23, 2011

I Will Figure this Out, Damn it!

...and she's sucked back in

One day I was at church, even though I'm not a church going person, I went with my family. The priest saying mass that day was an amazing man. His masses were always packed to the rafters. He was possibly one of the most enlightened priests I had ever known. During this particular mass he was talking about getting what you really want in life. He said, and I'm paraphrasing "When you talk with God and pray for what you want, be specific. If you want more money, tell him how much money you want. Don't pray in generalities. Pray with specificity." I remember his words really took me to my knees.

So in the last few days I have been thinking about some things. I was thinking about what it is that is holding me back from getting my perfect body. Why is nothing working? Because I am still living in a state of fear. I fear what I see in the mirror. I fear what the scale might reveal. I fear my current truth, and because I fear my current truth I cannot move forward. Isn't it funny that about a hundred chapters ago I stated that we have to accept ourselves the way we are now, but yet I haven't done this very thing. It is astonishing to me that I can sit here and absolutely know something intellectually, but I have been so programmed emotionally that I haven't been able to get to where I want to go. I am quite literally witnessing a battle between my intellect and my emotions.

I understood yesterday that fear was what was holding me back, and when I understood it, I immediately went out and bought a bathroom scale. It is time for me to face myself and accept myself for how I am today. It is time for me to understand the facts. It is time for me to go through the steps that I would normally go through when beginning a "diet." If we think about the steps to beginning a diet, there is some logic to it that works. The first thing that happens is we get sick and tired of being at the weight we currently are at. I know for myself, that every time I started a diet I would take a good look in the mirror and just get disgusted. Then I step on the scale to confirm my disgust. I don't think there has ever been a time when I didn't know exactly how much I weighed when I began a diet.

Here is the beauty in what's about to happen. I've done it before over and over; I just didn't realize I did it. I have lost weight many times in my life, but gave the credit to the design of the diet, or the quality of my commitment to the exercise program. What I never considered is that the entire time I was thinking thin thoughts, and as a result got a thin body. When I was a teen I didn't think thoughts of thinness or fat at all and I was slender. When I got slender while walking with my baby, I thought it was the walking. Instead it was the belief that I was becoming slender than made me slender. I have already done this time and time again, and didn't know it was my thoughts that were causing the thinness, not the diet or exercise.

Because I am really used to the structure of a diet and exercise plan, I'm going to design this new plan to mimic the diet and exercise thing. Now, truth be told, I have known for a long time that diets don't work, so I don't have to deal with that struggle. Let's look at what happens before, during and after a diet, and switch it up where necessary.

For me, what happens prior to the beginning of a diet, is hitting rock bottom. I believe I am there at 192.6 pounds. I am disgusted being at this weight, so this is my catalyst for change. So now I have decided to become a slim person. When I was dieting and exercising I always put "Abs & Workout" on my to-do list, so I've gone ahead and put it on there for me to check off when I've accomplished this task.

I used to get up early to do my exercising so I "got it over with" first thing in the morning, so beginning tomorrow morning I will get up at the crack of dawn. I will put on my mp3 player and listen to music while I sit at my computer journaling about being thin. In that journal I will write about how thankful I am that I finally understand these concepts, and thank the Universe for making me clear on this. I will be thankful for the speed with which I receive my perfect body and how the seventy-five pounds will just melt off my body. I will journal for a full half hour first thing in the morning, then go to my to-do list and check off "Abs & Workout."

Like when I was dieting I will weigh myself once a week to check on the progress of the fat melt, and celebrate when I see and feel it moving off my body. The rule of thumb is going to be when I have stopped losing weight for four weeks in a row, I am at the perfect weight for me, no matter what it is, and I can stop the diet. I will be slender for the rest of my life.

From this point forward I will come into this document and update my weight loss. Woo Hooo! Good bye seventy-five pounds. I'm going to call this The Diet to end all Diets.

October 30, 2011

One more time?

...punching my way out of a paper bag

I got on the scale and I gained two pounds. I've spent the morning contemplating the issue. I know there is an answer, and I know that the answer is simple. The fact of the matter is I've done it before but the problem is I've given credit where credit isn't due. I do think I have figured it out, although I wouldn't blame you if you didn't believe me or wanted to sock me in the mouth at this point.

Once again I went through the psychology of the diet and I'm laying it out here. I do believe I have put way too much emphasis on the mental portion of the equation and not enough on the physical. First, I'm going to make a blanket statement. You do not need to move your body to maintain your perfect body weight if you eat in moderation. I proved that as a young woman, and my mother also proved that. If you eat in moderation when you are at your perfect body weight you do not have to deliberately exercise. Movement makes your body stronger, and makes you overall healthier, but it is not necessary to maintaining weight.

With that said, most of us are not there. I believe that the reason that "diet and exercise" worked for me on various levels is this. First, I empowered myself by making a decision to be thin. Feeling empowered is much more positive than feeling like a victim. The next thing I did was take action. I always feel better when I am actively pursuing what it is I want, and in this case what it is I want is thinness.

So in essence I was absolutely right several chapters ago when I said that the last time I lost weight I had mixed results. I made a decision to be thin. I did not change my eating habits, but instead moved my body in ways that I enjoyed and in ways that I did not enjoy. I walked with my dogs with deliberate intent on losing weight and I did lose weight. I exercised my abdominals in a way I despised and I got a bad result.

The problem with the theories I have been working on is that they were not balanced. I have been preaching moderation and balance throughout this book, and yet I wasn't balancing at all. Because I felt that diets and exercise didn't work, I went full bore the other way, to the opposite extreme, using the power of my mind to control my weight, which is an out-of-balance way of trying to control a physical body. The mind and body have to work in concert.

Another thing I need to emphasize here, and cannot emphasize more strongly is you need to discover for yourself the amount of movement you require to start the weight falling off. Remember, my dog Lily can tucker herself out in fifteen minutes, but Riley can go for an hour. We all inhabit different imperfect bodies. What is right for me may not be right for you. One of the pitfalls we have taken on over time is a "one size fits all" approach to diet and exercise. A set amount of calories per person, amortized for males and females can't possibly work because we all have different needs. One person may burn faster than others. Eating in moderation for one person may be different than another. Different amounts of movement may be required for different people as well.

Try it for a week, if the weight begins coming off, then you have found it. If it isn't working, then move your body a little longer until it does work. This way you are balancing the food you eat with the movement to create the situation where the weight can just slide off easily.

So here is what I am proposing for the next week. Because I don't eat that much anyway, I do not need to moderate my diet. In fact to remind me that I am on a "diet" I am going to add some foods. I am going to add more fruit to my diet because I actually don't eat enough of it. I already know how much time per day I need to devote to moving my body in order for it to begin shedding pounds. I am resurrecting the bouncy ball dance party as my movement of choice.

Today is Sunday, October 30, 2011. In the tradition of a true diet, I will start tomorrow.

November 7, 2011

I'm giving myself whiplash, although I do make a very valid point here.

So far everything is going great. I have been doing a 40-45 minute bouncy ball dance party every day, and I have been enjoying the hell out of it. I look forward to doing it. My abdominal area is already firming up. I decided not to get on the scale right away because I wanted to truly replicate how I behaved in the past while on a diet. I never got onto a scale until it was so evident that I lost serious weight that I knew I'd be pleased with the results, so I am going to stick to that, although this morning I got better view of my feet, so that's encouraging.

Over the last few days I have been thinking about those pesky height/weight charts. You know the ones that say if you're 5'2" you must weigh 108 pounds. I have a serious problem with this idea, and needless to say I'm going to tell you why. First and most obvious, everybody is different. We come from different backgrounds. Today because of instantaneous travel and migration from one country to the next, we are mixing our genes up in a way that is unprecedented. Until the last few hundred years, those people born in one country lived their entire life in that country, had a family with people indigenous to that country, and then died.

The human form has adapted and evolved according to where it ended up living. In some areas of the world like colder climates, the body evolved into a larger, bulkier body to ward off harsh cold weather, and to endure the types of work that needed to be performed to survive. Look at tribes in Africa, the males are muscular on top but tend to be lean and sinewy in order to be able to hunt. A hunter needs the ability to run and run fast, so the African body type evolved into a sinewy one.

The European body is more average in nature (probably what the height/weight charts are geared toward) due to their penchant toward agriculture. The North American Body type was more like a cross between the African body type and the European, as Native Americans were both hunters and farmers.

The evolution of these body types took many thousands of years. Not only did body types evolve, so did skin color and texture, and hair.

The skin color and texture adapted to the environment it found itself in for greater survival of the species.

Now let's get to genetics. I'm no geneticist here, but this isn't really tough stuff to understand. Our genetic makeup is not limited to only the parents we were born from. Long lost genes are known to rear their heads when no one is looking. My husband has a patient who is short, dark and Mediterranean looking, and so is his wife, and they have a son who is six foot five and blonde. No one in the family is blonde, and no, parentage is not in question. Somewhere along the line the tall blonde gene just came rushing back out. We need to look no further than the Middle East to see evidence of the Crusades which took place more than seven hundred years ago. Most of the people in the Middle East who sport blue or green eyes probably have a female ancestor who was assaulted during the Crusades.

So between having genes from relatives who died centuries ago, and mankind's ability to move around the world and procreate with people from other cultures, there simply cannot be something we call normal. The minute we try to normalize or control this notion is the minute we lose control, and we have totally lost control.

November 8, 2011

...one foot on either side of the line

I do know I'm on the right track, but today I had another of my famous epiphanies. Over the weekend I viewed a two-minute video on You Tube. It was the actor Kevin Spacy being asked questions by students at a college. The student asked Kevin about how to endure the lean years while you wait for that career success to come. His answer was eye opening. I am paraphrasing him, but he said that success is not something external to you, it is inside of you. In order to be successful, you simply cannot desire that success. Desire alone does not allow it to come out. When you want to be successful at something you must have the desire, and also the talent.

You must teach yourself everything you need to know about what it is you want to do. You must learn from the masters. You must take action and control of guiding this desire into reality. Your passion must create it.

From Kevin's words, what I got out of what he said is that you create your desire with love and passion. This is true of everything in the world, everything. A man and a woman can have sex and therefore have a baby. If they are in love and are passionate about their relationship, they create a family, which is a higher order of things. My husband loves helping and nurturing people, and he is passionate about Chiropractic. He has morphed his love and passion into a six figure income. I say we apply the same principle here. I am calling it the Principle of Deliberate Creation.

Our success at losing weight is not external to us. The external would be Weight Watchers meetings, or diet pills or diet books. By reaching to the external we are saying that we are not responsible and someone better fix it. It is a crutch. By reaching to our internal love and passion, we will easily bring it to us. Let me show you how simple this concept is.

Love: I love being thin. Passion: I'm nuts about doing bouncy ball dance parties. Putting together the love with the passion is what will bring me back to my perfect weight.

November 10, 2011

On your mark, get set, go!
No matter what you read here, I do not grant permission.

I have good news. I figured it out for the last and final time. It took from June 3, 2010 to today for me to finally get here, but it is done. I have to say I'm pretty damn proud of myself. The final refinement to returning to our perfect natural weight manifested itself yesterday. Let me tell you what happened.

I went to work this morning, and then I went to run errands. All of a sudden I had all of these phone calls to make and answer, and demands put on my time. By the end of the day I realized I was supposed to learn something from all of this.

The lesson I got from it is that I do not have to have a bouncy ball dance party every single day to achieve my perfect weight. Convincing myself that this must happen every day is yet another rule, and there are no rules to being at your perfect weight. Everything in moderation. Everything. I am now doing bouncy ball dance parties every other day. I guess if you think about it this way, everybody loves a party, but would you really want to go to one every day? What makes parties so special is that you are rested and ready to go when they come up, and you enjoy them.

Back in the day when I would diet and exercise, I didn't exercise every day. I did it four or five times a week. It worked. Now I am going to do bouncy ball dance parties every other day until I am at my perfect weight. The whole idea here is to eliminate anything that feels bad. If I feel guilty because I didn't do a bouncy ball dance party, then that bad feeling is going to do more damage than any good the party would have done. I am tossing aside any feeling that is bad and going only with what feels good.

With that said I am granting permission to everyone reading this to go ahead and start having Bouncy Ball Dance Parties. I am only ten days in at this point but it is working like a charm. I feel my middle whittling down nicely.

I have determined for myself that between forty and forty-five minutes is enough, but honestly I enjoy it so much I have to convince myself to stop. More is not better, it's just more. Now as a warning, just so you know, when I get off the ball, my quads are a little shaky sometimes, but that's okay. I have been doing the parties for a while now and I have not experienced even the slightest bit of pain anywhere.

Like I said, this isn't for everyone, but for me I feel like I invented the most efficient and fun way to bring my body back. If you like it, great, do it. If you don't, find that body moving passion of your own. I absolutely do not write prescriptions.

I want to say thank you to my readers who have read my journey. I know this was convoluted at times and I was all over the map. I guess what I had to discover is that we as humans tried to control what it is that requires no control, only because we were striving to be something that we could not be, cookie cutter bodies conforming to one standard. If diversity is truly the goal, than we must accept that our bodies are also diverse, and perfect in that diversity.

It is my hope that those of you who have chosen to read this book will benefit from a shorter learning curve than I went through. I know that those of you who are older and have a longer point of view will probably be able to absorb the truth of this material faster than those who don't. Let us older people begin the revolution and show the younger set that these truths, that I have unfolded and reintroduced, are indeed the way. The struggle is over. Let's party.

November 23, 2011

Bouncy Ball Dance Party Perfection
They suck me back in and I tithe again too, and re-adopt The Cult language

It's been sort of bugging me that with all this time I've spent with the bouncy ball dance party, it didn't turn out to be what I had hoped.... that thing that would help us return to our perfect weights for the very last time. I thought maybe my criterion was too strict. My criteria for the perfect permanent slimming system is this: Low cost; fun; super-fast acting; non-time consuming. I mean come on, isn't that the opposite of a diet and exercise plan? That's what I really wanted, and I think a simple addition turns the bouncy ball dance party into the bouncy ball dance party-palooza!

This morning, in an attempt to make the BBDP more challenging, but still fun, I added one five-pound dumbbell. I started out the BBDP normally and danced with great enthusiasm, and then on the next song I picked up the dumbbell. I used the dumbbell the way you would use it on a flat surface, but did it while I was dancing. Curls, lat rows, shoulder presses, all of that stuff that we all know how to do but really don't like to do, okay me anyway. It became much more fun and easier to do when I combined it with music and dancing. Now here is the rub, just do it every other song. I did a half hour this morning, and I started and ended without the dumbbells, and the songs where I was using the dumbbells raised my heart rate and I did break a sweat.

With this system we are engaging the core, the heart and the muscle system all in one activity. You decide how much time you need to do this. What I believe just happened today was that I invented the single most efficient vehicle for returning to our natural weight. And remember, even if you don't like the weight part (you can opt to use two smaller dumbbells...one in each hand if you prefer). On my next round I am going to try using two smaller dumbbells and see how it works out. The true key may be using two smaller dumbbells and dance normally every other song. I'll get back to you later on.

I'm back again. I went ahead and refined the process and I think it might be perfect. Instead of one five pound dumbbell, use two two-pound dumbbells...one in each hand. Begin the party with a song and dance without a dumbbell (used to be called a warm up). Then alternate song to song using the weight. Dance normally, just with the weight in your hand. What you will find is that your heart rate increases and you actually break a small sweat. Make sure you end your party doing a song without the weight (formerly known as a cool down). This is now known as a bouncy ball dance party-palooza.

What I am recommending for myself is a daily bouncy ball dance party, but I bump it up to the palooza status every other day. The straight BBDP will wreak havoc with your belly. The muscles in the abdomen are greedy little critters and can be worked daily. I recommend palooza-izing your party every other day in order to rest those muscles that are being worked with the weights. You can additionally supplement with dog walks if you choose, but that is completely optional. I recommend a minimum of four parties per week, but if you are going to do the four, palooza-ize them all and put a day between each party. Forty minutes a day should do the trick, and you can even break that into two twenty-minute parties per day. Alright. That should be it. Winner winner chicken dinner!

December 1, 2011

....and she's back out again

I can see now what a hard time I'm going to have with my critics on this book. I've been all over the map.

Today while preparing a speech I will be giving, I went back to the book *The Secret*. I sat back and read the section about the body. Once again I must go back to my analogy about body temperature. It is truly the thoughts in our heads that determine our body weight. It is the beliefs, flawed as they are that pack on the pounds. I understand these concepts intellectually, and yet I once again tithed to the Cult. It keeps sucking me back in even now. I bought hand weights the other day. What a sucker.

The truth of the matter is that I am going to finally allow nature to take care of my body weight. Nature takes care of my body temperature, why not this? I have been so sucked in for so long that punching my way out has been awful. I have been doing some serious journaling today on the topic, and I have asked to be returned to my perfect weight of one hundred and eighteen pounds. I will sprinkle pictures of me at that weight around the house, and I even put in a request for expedited shipping. It is time for me to let go of the control that frankly I was bad at. My wanting to control my weight has resulted in my being seventy-five pounds overweight. I am releasing it to the world and letting nature take its course.

When I find myself being hard on myself for the state of my body, I am simply saying, "it is what it is...I did this to myself." But now I have hit the old ctrl+alt+del on my body to reboot to start fresh. I am defaulting to factory settings without any of my interference. It is time for my body to return to normal.

I believe this is going to work, now that I am relaxed and not feeling the need to control it. My first book, Unemployed is about to take off now. I have trusted the Creative Process to make this book happen big without my interference. I now trust the Creative Process to return my body to its natural state of perfect thinness at one hundred and eighteen pounds. It is not my job. It is my nature's job and I am finally going to let nature take its course.

While I was sitting here writing, I noticed a rubber band sitting on the table. I looked at the rubber band and it occurred to me that when you pull on a rubber band it stretches out, which is its unnatural state. However when you release control of the rubber band, it instantly returns to its natural state. By "controlling" my own weight, I have quite literally stretched my body into an unnatural state. By relinquishing control back to nature, I should snap back in record speed.

December 3, 2011

...and back into The Cult, but just a little bit

One of the things I have come to understand about attracting anything I really want into my life is to relax. Once I ask for it, if I relax it comes. This applies to ordering an item online. I don't sit around wringing my hands when I've placed an order for something I want. I just assume it's coming and move on.

One of the things I noticed about myself today is that I seem to manifest quite a bit of stress in my abdominal muscles. I am in such a near constant state of sucking in my stomach that it is ridiculous. When I was at my perfect weight of 118 pounds I never felt the need to suck in my stomach. Because I have focused so much of my negative energy concentrating on my stomach, naturally I have created these rituals to minimize the look, even though it doesn't do any good. I do know that being stressed is a very good way to keep away what it is I want.

To allow my perfect body to materialize it is time for me to make peace for the last time. Each time I feel my abdomen tense up, I am going to relax it. My body looks like it does because of the thoughts I have allowed inside my head. I will take an opportunity to relax my abdominals and to acknowledge how mean I have been to myself. I will look at the rubber bands on my wrist and know that my body is snapping back to where it once was before I blew it. I am relaxing and allowing my thinness to emerge. It is finally the time.

I've also found that I need to trick myself into thinking thin thoughts. I spend a tremendous amount of time focusing on the negative still. I am forever pulling up my pants and giving negative attention to my belly, at least hundreds of times a day. No wonder my belly is so huge. Today I bought a slimming camisole, not to make me look slim, but to make me feel slim. If I'm feeling fat I am powerfully attracting more of the same to me. If I feel slim I am going to powerfully attract more of that to me as well.

December 9, 2011

...and she is out for the last time...sort of

Today I had to review the video of my lecture at Rutgers University, and frankly it was painful. I felt thinner up there than I looked, so that was discouraging. I have the video up on You Tube for posterity, and proof that I was nearly two hundred pounds on December 5, 2011.

Today while I was journaling it occurred to me that I am still waging war on my belly. It astonishes me how I can know something intellectually, but have so much trouble accepting it emotionally. Way earlier in the book I said you really need to fall in love with yourself and come to a point of acceptance that your body is the way it is now. Yet I continue to abuse myself, and in particular, my belly. I am downright cruel.

While journaling this afternoon I wrote my belly a letter of apology. I don't pick on any other body part like I pick on my belly. I know my perfect state of weight will not come back to me until I truly made peace with myself.

I began looking at how I treated my belly as an abusive situation. No different than spousal or child abuse. I've been generally unhappy about my overall weight, but over the years I have just assaulted my belly with negativity. At one point my belly was my pride and joy, which probably explains why I have such anger towards it now. When I weighed my perfect one hundred and eighteen pounds my belly was perfectly flat and I never did a sit up. I would admire myself in the mirror and feel so good and happy. I loved how I looked.

Because I look awful I assault my belly like it's my victim. I say horrifying things to it, and now I'm strapped into an uncomfortable "slimming" camisole which only makes me feel worse. Yes it gives the illusion of feeling thin, but that isn't the answer, because once again, this method is coming from outside of me, and it needs to come from within.

While journaling I had a very long conversation with just my belly, and we declared a truce. If I stop abusing it with my words, thoughts, and this awful truss, my belly has agreed to relax and heal itself. Like all abusive relationships there has to be healing involved.

Another thing I have realized is that when I said that being overweight is a symptom, I was absolutely right. It is a symptom that I have been duped, lied to, and then allowed myself to abuse me. Intellectually and emotionally I have integrated the fact that I've been duped and lied to. I know beyond a shadow of a doubt that food has nothing to do with it, so I'm ahead of the game here. I have finally figured both intellectually and emotionally that moving the body has nothing to do with it. What I am trying to sift together now is forgiving myself for the torture I have allowed, and to let my body relax and begin the process of healing back to its default weight.

Whenever I feel negative attention go to my belly I am going to declare my love of my belly. I do remember the loving feeling I had when I looked in the mirror and saw that flat stomach. I know that flat stomach is in there. It is ready to emerge and my body is ready to normalize, now that I am doing the work to intellectually and emotionally completely understand this. I am ready.

I also read a wonderful quote on Twitter today, and I will attribute it to @templehayes: "Somewhere between the "no longer" and "not yet" is trust." I am no longer beating myself up, and I am not yet 118 pounds, but I trust I will be.

Ctrl+Alt+Delete...I am releasing **control**....I'm going an **alternate** route...I am **deleting** the weight.

December 28, 2011

...and she's out for good

Much earlier in the book, probably somewhere in the first twelve chapters I made a snarky remark about the "conventional wisdom" of losing more than two to three pounds per week being somehow dangerous, and how that seems so limiting. I visited the notion of losing a pound per day last fall, but then I dropped it. Yesterday a friend was talking about her "wedding weight loss strategy," as her daughter is getting married, and she commented that she shouldn't lose more than two to three pounds per week. It was all I could do to keep my mouth shut. This morning I got an email from a trusted source (which is why I opened it) touting yet another weight loss product that will allow you to lose a pound per day. All of this got me thinking.

I am here to say that a pound per day is not unreasonable, and I am here to talk about the perfection of losing one pound a day and how this is going to work. Science says it is unsafe to lose more than two to three pounds per week which is a belief based on limiting calories, and an exercise program. This has nothing to do with what I am proposing. We can lose much more than that per week and be perfectly healthy. Hell the fact that we are overweight is unhealthier than losing seven pounds per week.

I do believe I have the key here, and the beauty and simplicity are astonishing. Using the power of our mind, and assuming that we have managed to wiggle out of The Cult, we can lose one pound per day until we get to our perfect weight. Here is how we are going to do it starting today. I feel so strongly about what I'm about to propose, I am going to finish this book and begin the publication process. Okay, here goes:

Get on the scale and find out how much you weigh. I did and I am still at one hundred and ninety three pounds. In order to be at my perfect weight of one hundred and eighteen pounds, I need to lose a cool seventy five pounds. At one pound per day, that will mean that I will weigh one hundred eighteen pounds on April 10, 2012. After discovering the beauty of this I opened my journal and put on my headset and wrote about being one hundred and ninety two pounds today. If I am thinking it, it has to be my reality. I put on my headset and played music and journaled for twenty minutes about how happy and excited and grateful I was to be one hundred and ninety two pounds. Tomorrow I will journal about how it feels to be one hundred and ninety one pounds, and so on. What I love about this is that I am in no way, shape, or form controlling anything, but I am participating. Participating in the plan is important because it keeps your thoughts in line.

One of the things we will find is that knowing that one pound per day is do-able, allows us to get excited about how fast this is going, and it allows us to anticipate when we will see some results. For me this is key because there are always those doubts in the beginning of the diet because you don't see positive results for a few weeks, depending on how much weight you want to lose. Having the belief system firmly in tact is key to making this work. If you can't believe that you can lose one pound per day, you won't. Going through the motions without the absolute belief will not work. Completely removing yourself from The Cult is a must for this to work. Believing it will happen and journaling it into existence will allow your perfect body to come to you at record speed and with excellent health.

Also, what I'm finding helpful in keeping my emotions in check and neutralizing those negative thoughts about my abdomen is to make a statement in truth. When I feel a negative feeling about my belly, I make the following statement: Today I am one hundred and ninety two pounds and this is what one hundred and ninety two pounds looks like and feels like. Another statement in fact is that you already have your perfect weight. I may weigh one hundred ninety two pounds today, but within that one hundred and ninety two pound body is one hundred and eighteen pounds. So essentially my perfect weight has already arrived, it's just still in the box. It is a hard cold fact. My perfect weight is already here. This isn't wishful thinking, it is the truth. In the daily journaling you and I will be doing, we will briefly discuss the weight we are today, moving it down one pound each day. Be grateful for that weight for the day. Then turn your attention to allowing your perfect weight to emerge from your body. A visual that could be helpful would be like the peeling back the layers of an onion.

The one rule I will impose is that you turn your bathroom scale into a lovely centerpiece. Once you weigh yourself for the sake of getting clear, you are not going to get back on the scale until you are done, if ever. Back in the day, during the great rule of The Naturally Thin Empire, people did not own scales. If someone asked you how much you weighed, the answer always began this way: "Last time I went to the doctor..."

One of the things I know and have experienced for myself using The Principle of Deliberate Creation is that sometimes there is a time delay in getting what you want. For instance, if you begin as I did and journaled about being one hundred and ninety one pounds and use and feel all of the gratitude language, then step on the scale and I'm still one hundred and ninety three I'm going to get discouraged. It often takes a couple days to get things started, but it will start. Just put your head down and plow through it. Also remember if you have any doubts that this will work, it won't work. Depending on how much weight you have to lose you might not see any visual evidence for a long time. In my case I don't expect to see any real movement for at least four or five weeks.

This is where that quote I posted a couple postings ago comes into play. "Between no more and not yet is trust." We are no longer beating ourselves up and we are not yet at our goal, but in the meantime we trust that this is happening. If there comes a point where you know absolutely that it isn't working, you need to do an inventory of your belief system. See which belief is holding you back. If your entrenchment in The Cult is really severe like it was for me, you may want to consult with a coach that specializes in weight issues.

Another piece of advice I would like to pass along is stressing very strongly not to get on the scale. As we go from one day to the next journaling and talking about being one pound lighter you might not see this reflected on the scale or in the mirror right away. It has always been my history that I don't see any real change in my body for the first few weeks. Just keep doing it. When I did traditional diets, sometimes it was a month before I saw anything change, but when I did see change it was a lot of change. The scale is the tool of The Cult. Stay away from it. Just trust that the process is working. Remember it wasn't the diet or exercise plan that was dropping the weight all of those diets ago; it was your belief that was dropping the weight.

The beauty of this system is that there is no wishful thinking. I do absolutely believe that I will become one hundred and eighteen pounds one pound at a time, every single day. The feeling I have right now is the same one that I had when I began a diet and knew beyond a shadow of a doubt that this diet was going to work. It feels exactly the same.

January 31, 2012

After thirty four days of faithfully adhering to the plan, it didn't work. I believe the reason it didn't work, is that "one pound per day" is still me trying to control the show. As I thought this over these past few days, I realized that when I was actively dieting I didn't think about the weight I was currently at. I was only focused on the goal. The weight I was currently sporting made no difference to me. I had my sights set completely on the outcome. Outcomes are all that matters.

Back in the day when I committed to a diet and exercise plan, I had an immediate shift in my belief system. I believed that the reduction of calories combined with the movement of my body would result in a beautiful new body. I threw away the belief system that said I was a fat person, to an emerging thin person. As soon as I began the program, my thoughts immediately shifted from thoughts of fat to thoughts of how beautiful I was going to look. I didn't struggle with the shift, it was effortless. It was the shifting of the belief system that caused the beautiful body to emerge, not the diet and exercise plan.

This morning I found myself looking at Dr. Joe Vitale's work again in his book Instant Manifestation (2011). He references a technique that a friend of his Dan Barrett discovered called Remembering Your Future Past. Using this technique you actually begin an internal dialog as if your goal has already materialized. Dan said in Dr. Vitale's book "It's easier to remember than to create." In essence what I am trying to do here is create my perfect body using the power of my thoughts, just like I did when I thought it was the diet and exercise plan causing the weight loss.

This morning during a journaling session what I did was I wrote about how it felt the first time I saw some real results as my body began returning to normal. Here is a sample of what I wrote:

"I remember the day like it was yesterday. I had been working so hard for so long on this book and I was trying not to feel frustrated but I did. But that morning when I woke up, something felt different. Something felt weird. I could feel under the blankets that my body felt different. I sat up like a shot and felt my belly and it was flat. I mean flat as a board. I leapt out of bed and ran for the dresser mirror. I got up on tip toes and picked up my nightgown, turned sideways and there it was my flat belly. I hadn't seen that in thirty years. Wow. I turned to each side and looked, and then I went to the full length mirror, the one I had been avoiding all this time. I looked, and it wasn't a trick, my belly was flat and I looked great! That was the most awesome feeling in the world!"

Coming from a perspective of remembering evokes more positive emotion than asking for what you want. Wanting something automatically feels like you might not get that thing. Coming from a historic perspective indicates that you already have that thing. If you already have that thing, then certainly it must emerge. Allowing something to happen is much more powerful than simple wanting. Remember, in all likelihood you have already done this over and over and thought it was the diet and exercise plan. It wasn't, it was the shifting of your belief system, just like me.

So during my journaling what I'm going to do is talk about how it felt to feel my body changing and getting thinner. I have lots of experience because I've lost weight lots of times. When we diet we do think about how it feels to be thin. We do think about that a lot. So I am going to journal from the perspective of having already done it, and that my beautiful body is already here.

I have another concept to work with that may be tricky to accept but I am going to break it down for you. It falls under the category of "I already have it." Trying to pretend during the course of your day that you are already thin is rough. When you can't see it, you think it isn't there. This has been tricky for me too. It feels like a lie when I say stuff like "I'm a thin person" when in fact I look at myself and that isn't what I see. But let me see if I can turn this around a little bit.

As everyone knows I believe my perfect weight for my frame is one hundred and eighteen pounds. The fact of the matter is I already have it. I already have my one hundred and eighteen pound body plus seventy five more. So I can make the statement that my one hundred and eighteen pound body is already here, and be one hundred percent correct. Instead of losing weight what I am doing is allowing my one hundred and eighteen pound body to emerge.

So my approach from this point on is two-fold. For the sake of journaling, which I only do for about twenty minutes a day, I am going to write from the perspective of having already achieved my goal. To keep my thoughts positive, when I think about my body as I move through my day, the affirmation is "My perfect body is emerging" and variations of that theme. Also I will liberally treat myself to "I am" statements. If I can accept the notion that my one hundred and eighteen pound body is already here and is emerging, then the statement "I am thin" is actually true. If the conclusion to this book follows this page then I was successful.

I want to say thank you to my readers who have come on this journey with me. I know I was all over the map, but that is what The Cult has done to me, and how hard it was to come back to the truth. I apologize for the roughness of the ride, but I believe it was a necessary evil in order to get clarity on this issue that has been making me miserable for the last thirty years.

February 7, 2012

I was once again examining the phrase "The grass doesn't strain to grow," because on the topic of weight I do seem so fixated. I know intellectually that my declaration of intent of having my perfect one hundred and eighteen pound body is spot on, but I'm fouling up the follow through.

Here is where I'm tripping up the system. I fail to relax. I'm like a dog with a bone. I can't think of anything else but this. When I place an online order I immediately get a confirmation code and delivery date, and I don't think about it again. When I go on a diet and exercise program I have no idea how long it is going to take and don't give it another thought.

Up until now, I would do a journaling session daily just about getting back to my perfect weight. I was obsessively placing the order over and over again. If I doubted that the shoe store was going to fulfill my order and re-ordered the same shoes over and over, I would be over-run with too many shoes. I would get more shoes than I need or want. It's the same thing with my constant thoughts in my journal, and in my life about being the perfect weight. I am stressing and straining about an order that can't be delivered because I am screwing up with the shipping department.

When I was dieting and exercising I didn't send myself bad messages in my head because I knew absolutely that what I was doing was working. I knew with absolute belief. I thought thin thoughts when I exercised which sped things along, but I didn't really think about it after that. I am going to continue with the BBDPs and simply end the party with a slow song where I use the rubber tubing to gently address the other body parts that are getting slimmer and slimmer. Then I am going to leave good enough alone. No more journaling obsessively about my body. I am going to be that blade of grass once and for all.

February 8, 2012

I am not damaged goods. I am just healing from the abuse I've taken over the years. I realized today that clinging to the BBDPs and the rubber tubing is still going to the external. If I am going to go to the trouble of putting out a book on this topic I have to do it right. If I so much as rely on a party or do any exercise whatsoever, I am going to be raked over the coals, and rightfully so. I have to get over this hump. I have rejected The Cult completely. I have to have the intestinal fortitude to trust the creative process. I deliberately create things all of the time. I create on a daily basis.

When I wrote my first book *Unemployed* I knew that if I trusted the process the book would do what it needed to do without me stressing about it. I have been true to this, and I now realize that *Unemployed* and its sales are going to launch when this book launches. I know that nothing is going to happen with *Unemployed* until I get this book right. I have not wavered for one second or caused myself stress because I know in my heart that if I allow things to progress naturally they are going to hit the stratosphere. I have put all of my hopes and dreams into trusting the creative process because I see it working day in and day out.

Yet, since I turned the corner and swapped out my belief system on December 28, 2011, the one thing I haven't done is to relax and trust the process as it comes to my body. I believe it for everything else, but letting go and relaxing on the topic of my weight has eluded me. I wouldn't blame you for not believing me at this point. I realized that the journaling for my perfect one hundred and eighteen pound body every single day just reset the clock back to day one. I was placing the order over and over, which resets the clock for delivery.

Today when I journaled, I spoke of how nice it is to be thin. I said thank you for the body I'm in now. I said thank you for my new normal body. I reviewed my different body parts and wrote about how nice it is to have them be and feel thin. I spoke of thinness to myself very much the same way I did when I was dieting and exercising. I realized that when I was dieting and exercising, I was relaxed on the topic of weight because I had already declared to the Universe that I wanted to lose weight, and I thought quite a bit about being thin. When I would walk I would think thoughts about how the walking was making me thin. The Universe didn't hear the "walking" part, but heard the thin, because thin was the intention. I had given over responsibility for my thinness to the diet and exercise. What I had actually done was release control and allowed my body to begin returning to its natural weight. I just didn't know it.

I now understand that all of those times I did lose weight was not because of the diet or exercise, it was simply relinquishing control. Like my rubber band analogy, as soon as I released control and eliminated the stress of the control, the rubber band, and in this case, my body was able to easily and quickly snap back to its normal state. I am not going to depend on the BBDPs or the tubing. I am simply releasing control for the last time and let nature take its course. It is my job to get my ego out of the way, and allow nature to take its course. It is time for me to go into a state of absolute belief and trust that my body is returning to its normal and healthy state. My weight is not my job.

February 11, 2012

Being overweight can be based in your emotional life. The weight is never going to come off and stay off if emotional issues are causing it. Two days ago I got on a thought path about the state of my stomach and how I just never feel good and haven't for a long time. I picked up Louise Hay's book *You Can Heal Your Life* to see what these stomach issues may mean to me emotionally. Interestingly it meant that I was in fear of things changing (2004, p. 201). I thought that was interesting because I am a huge fan of change. I was somewhat perplexed by this.

I did some deeper thinking about what this means to me, and I came to realize that I wasn't concerned about changes that are coming in my life right now, instead this was an old fear I had been hanging on to all of my adult life. While I am not going to divulge what that fear was and who it involved, it is far too personal for me to talk about here, I will say that when I released that fear my stomach immediately felt better.

So I decided to poke a little further and looked up the terms "Fat" and "Overweight" in Louise Hay's book, and I was truly astonished. It was defined as "Fear, need for protection. Running away from feelings. Insecurity, self-rejection. Seeking fulfillment. Fear may be a cover for hidden anger and a resistance to forgive (2004, p. 169 & 189)." Several of these applied to me. I sat down with my journal today and talked extensively about those things that I have pushed away because they were too painful for me to deal with. I talked about circumstances that caused unbearable pain. I spent hours confronting the anger and the fear and the unfairness of certain situations that took place in my life more than thirty years ago. I realized that the spiral into my overweight began with some extremely painful events, and then exacerbated by the lies and insanity of The Cult.

I have spent a good deal of time today doing a mental inventory of what I'm angry about and what I'm in fear of. While it wasn't a lot of things, it was a few that rooted into my psyche between the ages of eighteen and twenty-four years old. I began adding this layer of protection over me because of the anger and fear that I was experiencing. When I stopped actively feeling these emotions, they were still there, but lying in wait for me to wake them up. Today they woke up. While I journaled about the root of my anger and fear, I got myself into a high state of agitation. I was just really pissed about things that happened a long time ago. I allowed myself to feel the feelings of resentment, anger and rage. I told the Universe to go fuck itself a few times too. I told the Universe it was a piece of shit for letting the things that happened to me happen.

The point is I felt the rage and anger and resentment over these circumstances for the first time in a very long time. I felt them and I felt them deeply. I cried and screamed to get them out. I took responsibility for what was my stuff, and then forgave for the things that I couldn't control. Finally when I calmed down I was able to let it go. I was able to let go of the people who hurt and disappointed me when I realized that what happened said more about them than me. With that I was able to find a place of calm. I actually had to go back into those situations and feelings and allow myself to deeply feel them again before I could let them go.

I highly recommend you look at the time in your life when you began to put on the weight and see if there wasn't an emotional catalyst that could be contributing to how your body looks right now. The beginning for me was seething writhing anger and resentment, followed by a platinum membership in The Cult. If you can't do this on your own, you may want to seek some professional help from a therapist. A coach is good if your sticking point is surrounding your belief system. A therapist will help you identify the emotions that could be holding you back. I have a dear friend who told me point blank that she did this to herself. She no longer wanted to be attractive to her mate and she allowed it to happen. Our emotions are very powerful. Between what we feel as an emotion and what we believe is our personal truth when it comes to weight can produce all sorts of outcomes that we do not desire. Now it is time to produce the outcomes that we do desire.

February 16, 2012

Since yesterday I have been thinking a lot about the state of disease versus the state of ease. When we live in a state of disease, our bodies are out of rhythm with nature. Nature and earth have a very predictable rhythm, and I know for myself that I am not in concert right now. Before I reveal how it is I am not in concert and how my perfect weight will not come back to me until I am in concert, let's examine what it is to be in a state of ease or a state of disease.

From Dictionary.com: The definition of dis-ease:

A disordered or incorrectly functioning organ, part, structure, or system of the body resulting from the effect of a genetic or developmental errors, infection, poisons, nutritional deficiency or imbalance, toxicity, or unfavorable environmental factors; illness; sickness; ailment. Any harmful, depraved, or morbid condition, as of the mind or society.

From Dictionary.com: The definition of ease:

Freedom from labor, pain, or physical annoyance; tranquil rest; comfort; freedom from concern, anxiety or solicitude; a quiet state of mind: Freedom from difficulty or great effort; facility: Freedom from financial need; plenty: freedom from stiffness, constraint; or formality unaffectedness: To free from anxiety or care: to mitigate, lighten, or lesson: to release from pressure, tension, or the like; to render less difficult: Facilitate.

This seems pretty obvious to me. Society as a whole on the topic of weight is in a state of dis-ease. Back when I was a child society was in a general sense of ease. Look at how many times in the definition of "ease" the word "freedom" was used. The word freedom does not appear one time in the definition of "dis-ease." The most important sentence in the definition of dis-ease is "Any harmful, depraved, or morbid condition, as of the mind or society." This fully and completely describes where we are as a society on the topic of weight. That is the definition of "The Cult."

February 19, 2012

When I coach clients on various issues in their lives, I tell them to pretend as if this thing that they want has already materialized. On the surface that seems sort of ridiculous. It isn't easy to pretend that it has already happened, but in the case of what I'm trying to do here it is essential. There are cool ways to trick the brain. I call it "behaving as if." Let's look at this process in a way that is familiar.

When a woman gets pregnant, generally speaking, she knows right from the beginning. In the beginning she can't see her baby, heck she can't feel her baby either, but she took the pregnancy test and sure enough the baby is in there. Now anyone that has been pregnant will know that once you get a positive test result you don't keep taking pregnancy tests day after day after day. Once it is known that you're pregnant, you begin behaving as if. You take prenatal vitamins and go to the doctor regularly to make sure all is well. As the big day comes closer and closer you paint the baby's room and begin gathering items that you need in order for the baby to be comfortable and for your role as a parent to go smoothly. If you are really lucky your family or friends may throw a baby shower for you to help you get the things you need. By behaving "as if" you have guaranteed that when the baby arrives you are ready for the event.

The same thing goes with The Principle of Deliberate Creation. I ordered my perfect body a long time ago, so I don't need to go through that exercise yet again. It is already out there. I have rejected The Cult, so I can check that one off the list as well. By relaxing and giving over the responsibility back to nature, I am in a calm state. I know that this is going to be done. Now it is time for me to behave as if my perfect body is already here.

Yesterday I went to the store and bought myself a bra in the size I was when I was one hundred and eighteen pounds. This may sound like I'm turning my back on buying clothes in the wrong size. Actually that would be true. In the past I would buy clothes in the wrong size hoping that I would lose weight. Hope, like trying has a failure option. Now that I am at the point where I am absolutely certain this is going to work, I am treating myself to the types of clothing that I have not squirreled away for when I finally get thin. Those are already in my closet. Literally I have a closet full of clothes that I will be able to wear moving forward. However, I have not purchased intimate apparel, so I am starting with that.

In order to behave as if, I went up to my bedroom and inventoried my closet. I almost have nothing left to wear so this needs to work pronto. I rearranged my closet so that the small clothes are in the front ready to wear. I cleaned out my dresser drawers so that they can be ready for the smaller clothes that I will be wearing shortly.

The Universe loves gestures, and moving these clothes around and buying something special and new every day is a powerful message to send to get this thing going. Tomorrow I am going to move a full length mirror into position to be able to see my beautiful new body. You might be asking yourself how long this is going to take. I have no idea, but the more prepared I am the more I am sure that I will return to my perfect weight in record time. The Universe loves speed and loves to deliver when the recipient is ready.

It is not up to me to determine how long this process will take. Because I have completely rejected The Cult, I do not have to be wrapped up in the limiting behaviors that say I can only lose two to three pounds a week. My body is free to return to its perfect weight as quickly as it would like. The only thing I am concerning myself with is outcomes. The only thing that matters is having a tunnel vision of the outcome I want and let nature take care of the rest. The speed is none of my business, although I must admit I'd like it to come quickly.

So in the end, once you can absolutely reject the teachings of The Cult, and I mean completely and utterly reject it, you can turn the corner like I have. Reject The Cult. Relax and understand that you aren't in charge and you never have been, nature has. Decide on what weight is right for you and have tunnel vision to get there. Get really excited about it, like you placed an order for the best thing you could ever have purchased. Be grateful for what you already have. Be grateful for the body you have today because that body is going to morph into the body you will love looking at and exist inside of. Be in a state of gratitude for what you already have and let the good news that your perfect body is returning allow you to catapult into a state of joy.

The Universal Intelligence, which is accessible to all of us, feeds on our positive energy. When we are in a state of negative energy, nothing good can happen. In the last fifty years we have gone from a state of serenity on the topic of weight, to a desperate situation which is based in fear and stress. It is time to look at the outcome that we want for our bodies. Not to look like someone else's body, but to be happy and content in the body we were born in. It has been so long since we were content to be in the bodies we were meant to be in, that when it happens we will be truly content, and that, in and of itself is a miracle. It was the desperation to look like someone we can't look like that started this problem. Let us end the problem by being content to be in the bodies we were born into.

February 21, 2012

The final key in allowing your body to return to its own state of perfection is to relax. You see when we are in a state of "trying to lose weight" this implies that there is effort on our part to do it. If there is effort involved, there is also stress. Stress will keep the weight on. There will never be a perfect outcome if you are in a perpetual state of trying. I heard it once said that "trying is failure with honor." Or as Yoda from Star Wars said "Do or not do, no try."

In my case, I have asked. I asked a long time ago and I don't need to ask again. I am well aware of exactly how much I want to weigh. I do absolutely believe that I will return to my state of natural thinness, and it will happen quickly. Now it is my turn to completely relax knowing that this is coming. What I've been doing on an emotional level up until now is equal to placing an order online, and then be in a constant state of running to the door to see if the package arrived yet. This is too much high level stress. It is time for me to move on to another topic for another book and just allow this to happen.

The topic of my next book is the state of health that we find ourselves in this world. It is time to unleash what I have discovered when it comes to weight, onto the topic of disease. Using the Principle of Deliberate Creation, I have cured my own high blood pressure, raised the serotonin level in my brain, and most recently cured a long running stomach ulcer. As I approached my level of stress today as it comes to the topic of weight, I realized that when I actively decided to cure these diseases using the power of my mind, one of the most important factors was when I did it I was in a state of complete relaxation.

Allow your mind to relax, but also relax your body. I suck in my stomach all of the time, and this is a stress response. Today I relax my body and allow it to return to normal.

October 3, 2012

Since the last entry I continued to struggle. Some interesting and mind blowing things began to happen to me. My daughter was getting married, and I put off getting my dress for as long as I could. It was the fear of being measured and having to face it that was holding me back. Finally, under duress, and after a very long crying jag I went and did it.

The seamstress who measured me said I was between size twenty-two and twenty-four. I told her to order the smaller size because "I'm losing a lot of weight." I made this statement quickly and fairly flippily. My entire motivation was to get out of the shop as fast as I could. I was having a bad day and this was only making it worse for me. When I got in the car I vowed that I would NEVER EVER cry over my weight again. I was done.

In July my dress came in and I had to go for a fitting. I wasn't looking forward to it at all. I went to the shop and they brought me the dress. When I put it on I looked like I was playing dress-up with my mommy's clothes. The seamstress came in and asked me point-blank who originally measured me because they did a lousy job. I told her that she measured me. I had clearly lost about 2-3 dress sizes.

I believe the weight came off for two reasons. First, I faced my fear and vowed never to let it happen again. Second, I made the statement 'I'm losing a lot of weight" which set the wheels in motion for the weight to come off. The simple act of saying that I am doing something made that thing happen.

While I was happy that I had lost weight, I immediately began stressing about how I was going to look in the dress, being that I was mother-of-the-bride. I became uncomfortable with how I looked and couldn't be grateful for the weight loss that I had. I began worrying that the dress might not fit. I stopped losing weight at that point.

For the next two months I kept reading the passage about weight from the book *The Secret*. I also read more from Louise Hay's book *You Can Heal Your Life*. In *The Secret* Rhonda Byrne says to "think thin thoughts" and Louise Hay said to make "I am" statements. I came up with "I am thin" but that didn't feel right because I'm not. Finally yesterday I got to the bottom of it. I once again inspected the emotional side of dieting and realized that a diet begins with a decision. The decision is made to lose weight. Once that decision is made, the negative thoughts about our bodies disappear and are replaced by thoughts of losing weight. The statement we make to ourselves is that we are on a diet and we are losing weight. We remind ourselves of this all day as we make special foods and do special activities that we believe are causing the weight loss, but they aren't causing weight loss at all.

It isn't the special foods or activities; it is the thoughts about weight loss that cause the weight loss. Yesterday I sat back and thought about what happened between May and July with my weight and I knew it was simply the utterance of that one statement in the bridal shop that got the ball rolling. It was my anxiety that caused it to stop. I am now completely and absolutely calm and know that the weight is coming off easily and quickly because I finally figured it out.

I have also found that the Universe likes speed. Making statements like "I am losing weight quickly" is far more powerful than the statement "I'm losing weight." In physics, things are measured in speed, not time. Even many of our body functions are measured in rate and speed, like heart rate and breathing rate. Time is a man-made convention. It is necessary for the function of the day, but it isn't how things are measured in the Universe. The Universe does not understand time, but it does understand speed. We measure light in speed, and we measure sound in speed. Making the statement over and over in our heads "I am losing weight quickly" is extremely powerful. We made these statements to ourselves over and over every single time we dieted. You said to yourself and others "I'm on a diet and I'm losing weight" and that is what caused the weight to come off. It is when you worried about the ending of the diet and the weight coming back, that the weight came back.

Look at it this way; we are a product of two entities, the conscious and subconscious. I am going to call this our Youniverse. In our Youniverse, the conscious is the master and the subsconscious is the servant. The master makes the demands and the servant carries them out. If you are saying "I am losing weight very quickly now" the servant has no choice but to carry it out because you have declared it to be so.

The servant obeys exactly what you tell it to do every time exactly the way you say it. This goes, not only for your weight, but for everything in your life. You speak it and it is so in your Youniverse.

I have also noticed, when I added speed to the thought, I began feeling the weight coming off. In little patches all over my body I feel a tightening. It is a momentary feeling and it moves around. This is nature's way of telling us that the process is underway. When we lost weight the old way, by believing that it was unhealthy to lose more than 2-3 pounds per week we couldn't feel the tightening because the process was moving too slow. I mean I drive a Jaguar and I can hardly feel the car moving when I'm going twenty-five miles an hour, but when I put the pedal to the metal, the car roars and takes off like a shot. This is no different.

So here it is in a nutshell. Declare that you are on a D.I.E.T. This stands for "Do It Effortlessly Today." Tell yourself that you are losing a lot of weight quickly. The process will start immediately. You will feel the tightening of your body parts. You don't even have to believe it to get it started. Remember, I made one simple statement that I didn't necessarily believe in the bridal shop and eight weeks later I had lost about three sizes. It was the combination of the statement and the relaxation on the topic that allowed me to slim down. Belief that the process is working is not necessary....just get started.

The one thing that will stop the process is fear. If you continue to wring your hands and cry about your body you will not lose weight. When we used to diet we got excited about knowing that we were about to get thin. This is the process that started it, not the deprivation of calories or the grueling exercise. It was the thoughts and the excitement around the thoughts. Remember if you add speed to your statement it become so much more powerful, you will actually feel your body reshaping itself.

We can deliberately stop the process of losing weight as well. Once we return to our perfect weight, the thoughts go from "I'm losing weight quickly" to "I'm thin." That's it. Once we get there we will never have to lose weight ever again. The "I'm thin" statement will eventually become a part of who we are until we don't have to utter anything to ourselves about our bodies again. It will just be. The absence of thought will default the perfection of our bodies. Just like how our bodies regulate our body temperature without thought.

Okay, for the last time, I am finally done. I did it. It took twenty-eight grueling months, to the day, to work this problem out. I am so glad to be finished. Now onto the next book while I let nature take its course and slim me down to my natural weight. Oh readers we did it! I couldn't have done this without you. Now let's all go and grab us some skinny! I love you!!!!!!

February 2, 2016

"In case I don't see ya, good afternoon, good evening, and good night." – Truman Burbank as portrayed by Jim Carrey—The Truman Show 1998

It has been three years since I have written a word in this book. Something was still bugging me and I was still fat. A lot has happened in the time since I began writing this book nearly six years ago. My oldest child, my daughter has gotten married, and is now a mother herself. My darling grandson is the light of my life. We have moved to a new town, into a home I have only dreamed of. I am teaching College Success at my alma mater, Union County College, which I love teaching more than I can express. So essentially, since the last entry into this book, my life has taken a turn for the better. I am exponentially happier.

In the last three years I have spent countless hours re-dissecting the events between the fittings for my dress for my daughter's wedding. I knew the final answer took place in that time period, and whatever it was that happened, was the simple fix I was looking for. In the years since that time, I have studied with great focus on how the mind/body connection and The Placebo Effect can make drastic changes in human health. While I originally published this book in frustration, I knew I wasn't done, and knew in the deepest recesses of my soul that I wouldn't quit until I figured it out. No one was banging at my door to get to the book, so I knew time was on my side.

Today I decided to re-edit the book and to look at those specific items that I knew were working. There were many concepts I lay out in this book that, when I look back at them, were actually quite intuitive. Here are the things that ring absolutely true, and then I will conclude with the ridiculously, stupidly, insanely simple solution to returning to our ideal body weight. Batten down the hatches readers. I swear on my grandson's head this time. I'm really done.

- Fall in love with yourself. It feels amazing when you fall in love with someone else, so do it for yourself. Besides, no one is better than you. The entire key, the ENTIRE KEY to all of this, is feeling good.

- Use your emotions, not your thoughts, as your guide
- Visualize happily the body you want
- Meditate...it is so good for you emotionally as well as physiologically
- You are not losing weight, you are defaulting to factory settings...you are returning to normal
- <u>Knowing</u> it is happening, quite simply, allows it to happen
- The complete absence of thought or belief returns your body to balance
- If you are overweight your beliefs are simply out of balance. It is not the crisis The Cult makes it out to be. It is simply an indicator. You are feeling bad more than you're feeling good. Just like running a temperature is not an indication of impending death, it's just information that says something is going on here.

Of these eight items, all of them are based in feelings and emotions. Even the absence of feeling is a neutrality that our body responds to. When there is an absence of feeling or belief system, the body returns to balance because it is not being interfered with or experiencing resistance. **Negative thought is the resistance that stops what you want from coming to you, no matter how hard you try.** The human body is designed to always be seeking balance, or homeostasis, and resistance of any sort negates that balance.

The process of weight management that we have invented and embraced since the 1960's begins with a feeling of negativity about our body. It can't work when it begins with negativity. Then we treat the negativity by eating foods we don't like and exercising in a way we don't enjoy. We try to manipulate a negative with another negative. Didn't mom always say "two wrongs don't make a right"? This system of negativity cannot and does not work long term. But it does work in the beginning, which is why this process has hung on so long.

The reason why it works in the short term is because initially we get excited. We feel like we are doing a good thing for ourselves and we get all excited by launching rockets of desire. With that excitement and anticipation, our bodies pump positive, naturally occurring endorphins such as oxytocin, serotonin and dopamine. What we are doing is breaking the negative feedback loop of our own untrue and negative beliefs about ourselves through activities that release excellent chemicals that allow us to feel good for hours after the effort is over.

As time marches on, and finally the evidence comes that all of this hard work is paying off, our good feelings morph into true excitement as we look in the mirror and love the image we see. Then the weight comes off even faster and faster. This happens until an inevitable screeching end. Because we have put the responsibility for our achievement on the diet and exercise plan (rather than our positive emotional mindset), when we can no longer keep it up because it is boring and uninspiring, our minds snap back to the negative emotion of gaining weight. When we are no longer feeling good, we crawl back to our old cozy belief system, and the weight returns. We are simply vacillating between two belief systems that feel shitty. We are in a never ending loop of feeling awful with tiny little shards of good feeling in the middle. This is where yo-yo dieting comes from.

People who are permanently successful on traditional diet and exercise programs tend to make all or part of the process a permanent part of their life. They may be the few who find their way to feeling good all of the time doing what they do on the diet and exercise plan, because they actually enjoy it. Statistically speaking there will be some who love it and succeed. However, most of us feel extremely restricted by this.

When we decide to diet, the first thing we feel is a sense of relief because <u>we know for a fact it will work,</u> and the responsibility is off our shoulders for the first time in a long time. On the continuum of good feelings, relief is on the bottom, but that's okay. It may be on the bottom, but it makes the grade of a positive emotion. It is a place to start. Then as time rolls on, we feel better and better. When we add moving our bodies, we release those wonderful natural pharmaceuticals that help us break the negative feedback loop. For most of us, the negative feedback loop is so completely automatic, we don't even know we are thinking the thoughts and feeling the emotions that are making us miserable. We have been so trained by The Cult to whip ourselves over every little "transgression", we don't even know we are doing it. Luckily we have super heavy duty chemicals at our disposal. We have our own personal brain pharmacist.

As it turns out, what happened to me between dress fittings was simple. I left the shop and went out to my car and declared out loud, that I would never allow myself to feel that way again. I said "I am losing a lot of weight and doing it quickly" to the seamstress just to get me the hell out of there. My subconscious took that as a command and ran with the ball. Once I pulled out of the parking lot I was in a state of complete relief. You have to understand, I had worked myself up into a pretty thick lather about being measured for this dress (one of the most important dresses a woman will ever wear), so simply having it over with, regardless of the outcome, was a huge relief.

A few interesting things happened once I got home. First, I felt much better. Then I went back to my twice daily bouncy ball dance parties. I had no hope of losing weight at that point and I wasn't even trying. I just really enjoyed doing the parties. I danced about twenty minutes twice a day and when I finished I felt really happy and good. I didn't consider it exercise, because frankly it isn't. I just felt good, and it felt good to feel good. Moving my body during a bouncy ball dance party was enough to release those chemicals that brought on the good feelings. Doing it twice daily spread that chemical sensation throughout the day which was awesome. I felt better than I had in months. The final piece of the puzzle would be what I tell my college students to do, and that is to let it go (private note to my UCC101 students...eat a sandwich). Finally, I was so distracted with the wedding plans that I didn't really have time to think about my waistline. It wasn't until after the second fitting that I promptly destroyed all of the good I had done by worrying about being fat again.

So here is the bottom line on how to return to your natural ideal weight. Decide that this is what you want. Put a number in your head and keep it there. Feel the relief of a good decision and launch that rocket of desire. Now move your body in any way that you like so those delicious pharma-goodies rain all over your brain making you feel crazy good. Eat whatever you want, but do so in moderation. The human anatomy doesn't like too much or too little of anything. It likes balance.

Reach for a better feeling emotion whenever you can. Don't worry about your words and thoughts. Read your emotions. Distract yourself. Do things that keep your mind positively occupied and off your waistline. I am learning how to speak French, and I listen to audio books. Let it go. What we have been taught by The Cult is the opposite: Hang on and obsess over it constantly. This is a recipe for mental illness. Like I said in an earlier chapter, it is nothing but a case of SWAD (Social Weight Anxiety Disorder), and the easiest way out is to tap the pharmacist in your brain and get some of those juicy drugs flowing in your system, but this time on your own terms, and the way you like it.

I am not saying that you will go from feeling like crap to being Pollyanna...it is a process after all. Getting fat was a process too. Start with relief and just keep reaching for the next better feeling up the ladder. The better you feel, the easier it gets. The easier it gets, the faster it comes. The faster it comes, the sooner you will be done with this forever.

We have been on a continuum of emotion that goes from feeling shitty to feeling crappy, when we thought we were on a continuum of feeling bad to feeling good. That is simply not the case. To break this once and for all, we must abandon the model where we go from feeling really shitty and applying really awful choices in order to elevate ourselves to feeling crappy; to instead, starting with a sense of relief and allowing ourselves to get better from there.

I began this chapter with a quote from the 1998 movie, *The Truman Show* starring Jim Carrey. The premise of this movie was the lead character, Truman Burbank, was born into a television series about his life. He didn't know that everything about his life was a lie. The people in his life were actors and the town he lived in was an elaborate television set. The show was on twenty-four hours a day, and people were riveted to see what Truman would do next, and to see how long it would take him to figure out that nothing in his world was real. It was the ultimate social experiment.

I feel like a real-life Truman Burbank. Six years ago, things just stopped making sense to me. I couldn't shake the idea that none of these weight problems we suffer with today were problems before. If we are charged with controlling our weight now, why were we not charged with controlling our weight throughout the history of time? Why? Because it is a fiction. It's simply not true. Nature wouldn't do this.

Wish me luck. I will be called every name in the book. There will be a feeding frenzy calling for my head. Hopefully with time, cooler heads and common sense will prevail, because to boil things down, this is a simple matter of common sense. Nature likes simplicity and what humans have done is create a situation of such mass complexity, it was bound to collapse under its own weight eventually. Pun intended

Conclusion

I am in no way a scientific expert on this topic. I'm just a regular person who felt like something was totally wrong and I was frustrated as I embarked on this journey. I knew that somehow, some way, we were completely missing the boat and ignoring the fact that life ending overweight was never a widespread issue in our human history, and yet no one was talking about that. I knew this had to be the pathway unexplored.

As I stated early in this book, people have looked for ways to reduce their weight and change their appearance for at least the last two hundred years or so. I am not in any way trying to suggest that vanity is a new phenomenon. Prior to the 1960's women's magazines were littered with advertisements for trusses and girdles, and on the very back pages were ads for different tonics that promised slimmer bodies. The advertising in men's magazines was for gadgets to get guys to look like Charles Atlas, a body builder in his day. As long as there were people who wanted to be thinner or wanted to change the appearance of their bodies, there were snake oil salesmen to step in. Today it is no different, other than the fact that snake oil salesmen believe what they are selling because they have "science" on their side. Yet the "science" changes and contradicts itself daily and no one has screamed "STOP!" until now.

In the mid 1960's weight was not a medical issue. It was not a social issue. Because the vast majority of people accepted their bodies as they were, bodies tended to be normal. If you don't believe me, take a look at any picture taken in a busy street scene prior to the 1970's or so. Not a fat or obese person to be found. Of course they existed because humans come in all shapes and sizes, but it wasn't normal by any stretch of the imagination. Today being overweight is normal. It is absolutely normal. It is more than normal. It is expected. There are two generations who never saw what normal is really like. This is terrifying.

What happened in the 1960's was a trifecta of epic proportions. Three major influencers rose to prominence simultaneously: Science, Media and Business. Science, and more specifically, medicine, began coming into its own in the 1960's. Medical doctors were looked upon as Gods who could do no wrong, by the average citizen. Medical doctors required enormous amounts of education and training when measured against the average worker of the time. Most people did not go to college back then. So, whatever the medical community reported to be true, was accepted without question by the public.

Business had grown to be the savior of society. The young adults of the 1950's and 1960's were born of parents who survived The Great Depression; World War II, and the Korean Conflict. Compared to what they had been through, business was offering jobs and products that made life easier. Companies and products were largely trusted by the consumer.

Then there is the media. The influence of media began to grow exponentially in the 1960's with regular daily viewing of network television, and on-the-spot reporting from the ground in Vietnam. The American public got their first look at what war really looks like from a television screen in their living rooms. Advertising also went from selling soap and cigarettes, to really forming the consumer's appetite for things. Advertising became extremely manipulative and used fear tactics to get consumers to make purchases. Fear tactics like having bad breath, or the dreaded "ring around the collar." Fear is the birth mother of The Cult.

Media also exposed the average American to images that would dictate our opinion of the human body from that moment forward. Images of women in magazines and on television who were either naturally very thin, or unnaturally very thin, but thin is what we got, and this became the standard of what women thought they had to be. Nature and common sense simply vanished.

The public bought the images and the science around losing weight as if these were coming directly from God. No one questioned the righteousness of the "information" being produced. So trusted were doctors that new information and new diet advice was readily consumed, even though over and over, throughout the decades, the "findings" have been routinely debunked by evidence.

Today, fifty years later, society is still clinging onto whatever science, media or business brings out to offer. You cannot hear a news teaser without some reference to a new study that claims that your houseplants or your fluorescent lighting is causing you to get fat. No one, at least no one I have heard of, has yelled "stop the madness!" until now. No one has looked backwards and said, "What the hell have we done?" No one has even remarked that none of this was necessary one hundred years ago. There is no fat disease. There is no fat virus.

Today there are studies being conducted by major universities and hospitals such as Mt. Sinai in New York that are looking at the influence of emotions on health. There are those innovators such as Deepak Chopra, M.D. who is straddling the line between modern medicine, holistic/eastern medicine (Ayurveda) and spirituality (meditation and positive psychology) in his research through The Chopra Center for Wellbeing and The Chopra Foundation. You can read more in his book *Super Genes* which he co-authored with Rudolph E. Tanzi, Ph.D. If you want to learn more about emotions, belief, brain functionality, and neuroplasticity, I highly recommend the book *You are the Placebo*, by Dr. Joe Dispenza. At some point, science is going to understand the direct impact that the emotional system has on bodily function, and this includes body weight. The evidence is already being published in peer reviewed journals.

The Limbic System is the part of the brain that is responsible for motivation, emotion, long-term memory, among other functions. It doesn't take a scientist to understand when the human brain is bombarded with negative messages, this is going to depress or repress at the very least, the Limbic System. Freeing us from the negative messages and allowing the Limbic System to work at its optimum is part of the process that releases the chemicals that allows us to feel good and healthy and vital. For the last fifty years the media, science and business have used fear tactics to repress the collective and individual Limbic System. We have all heard about people who died of a "broken heart." Their grief repressed their Limbic System enough to cause death. This is how powerfully our emotions effect our bodies.

It is time to turn the corner back into a positive mode to return our bodies to a normal state. It is also time to put the negative messaging to a humane sleep and allow us to function normally again without fear. Returning to our normal weight, sociologically will solve a plethora of problems that no one could have predicted fifty years ago when this all began. Imagine what the world will be like when millions of people will no longer be worried about calories or their weight. Imagine what problems will solve themselves, and imagine the time that will be freed up to solve the most complex problems of the world.

Perception is awareness shaped by beliefs. Beliefs "control" perception. Rewrite beliefs and you rewrite perception. Rewrite perception and you rewrite genes and behavior...I am free to change how I respond to the world, so as I change the way I see the world I change my genetic expression. We are not victims of our genes. We are masters of our genetics.

-Bruce Lipton Ph.D.
Cellular Biologist

About the Author

Laura Dolan-Hayes is a success coach, author, humorist, and college success professor who lives in Plainfield, New Jersey with her husband Ken and her many loving pets. She received her BA in Information Technology & Informatics, and a MA in Communication at the School of Communication & Information at Rutgers, The State University of New Jersey. Her first book *Unemployed: How Desperation Led Me to the Worst Job Ever* is available at book sellers' world-wide. You can find her on Facebook, Twitter, Instagram, and on her website www. successdolanhayes.com.

www.ingramcontent.com/pod-product-compliance
Lightning Source LLC
Chambersburg PA
CBHW051429280526
45785CB00003B/1219